Advanced Studies in the 21st Century Animal Nutrition

Edited by László Babinszky, Juliana Oliveira and Edson Mauro Santos

Published in London, United Kingdom

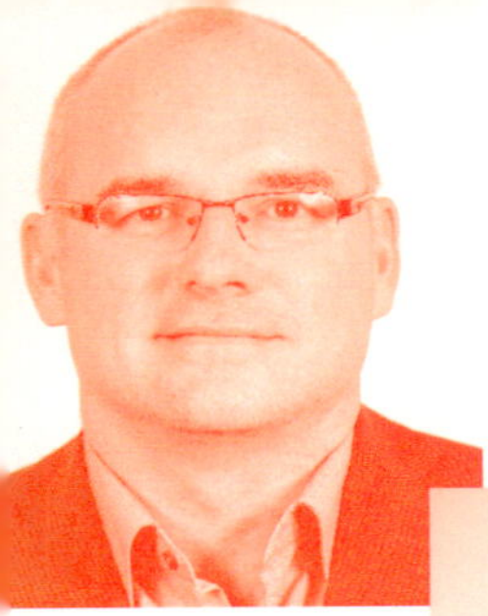
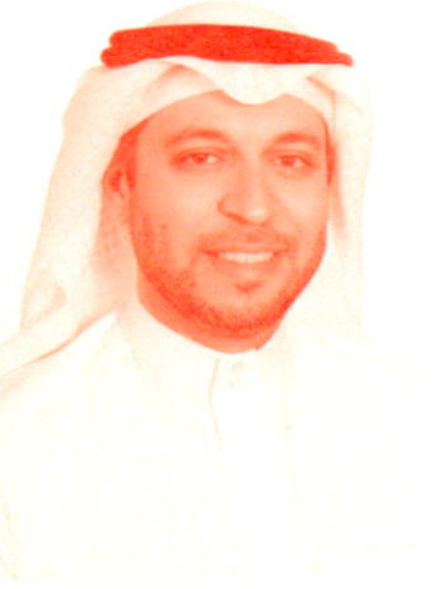
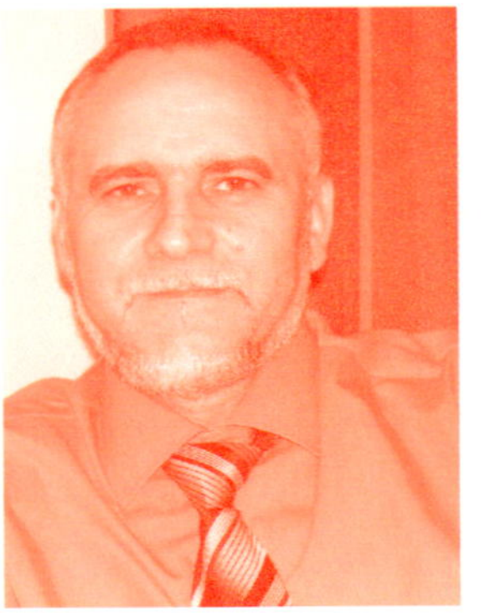
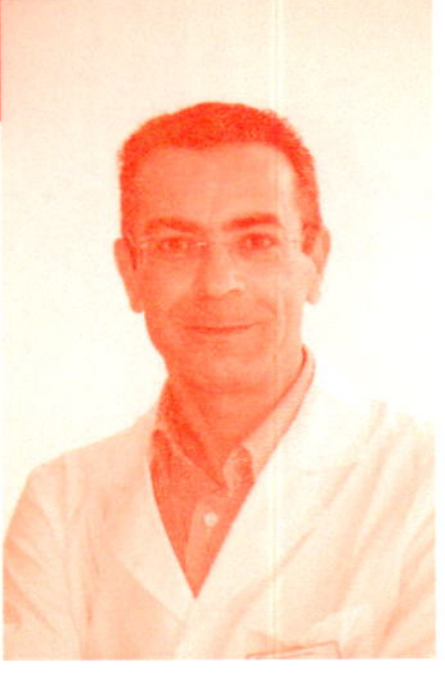
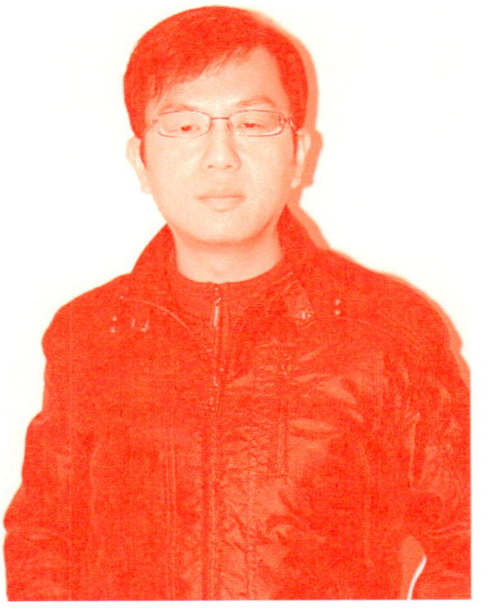
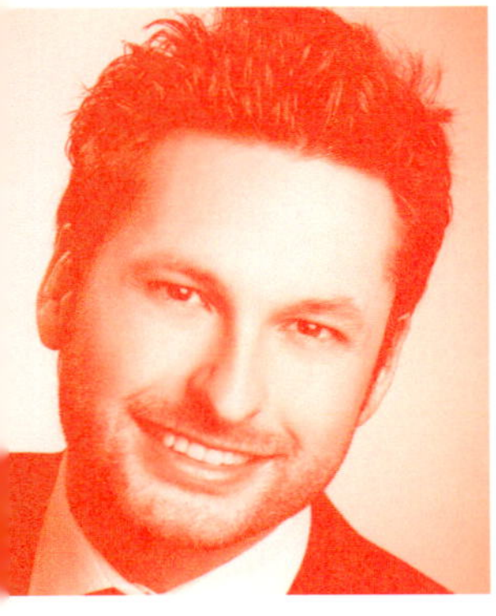
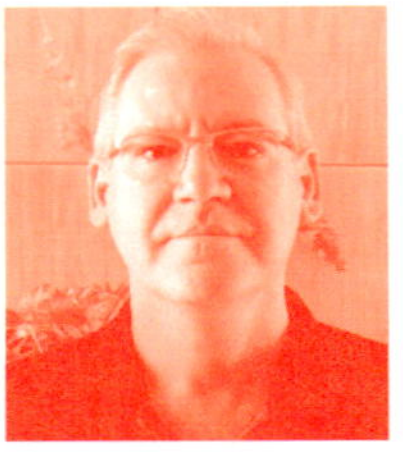

IntechOpen

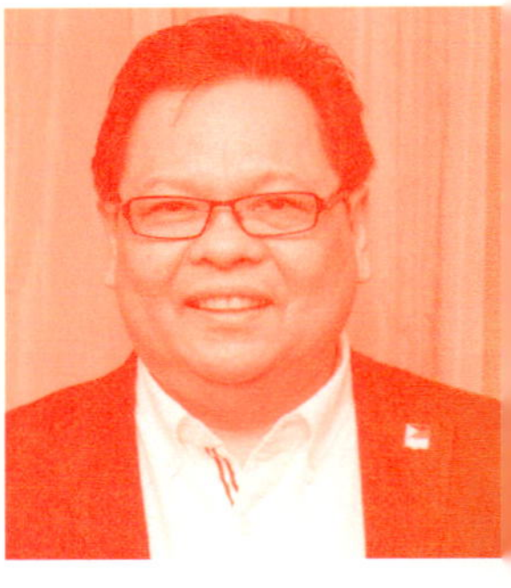
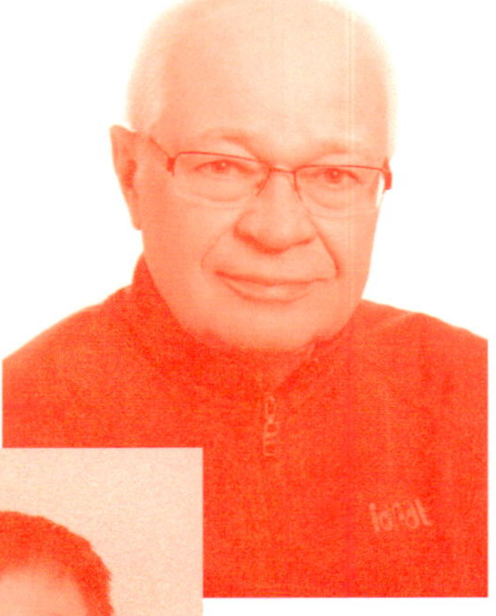
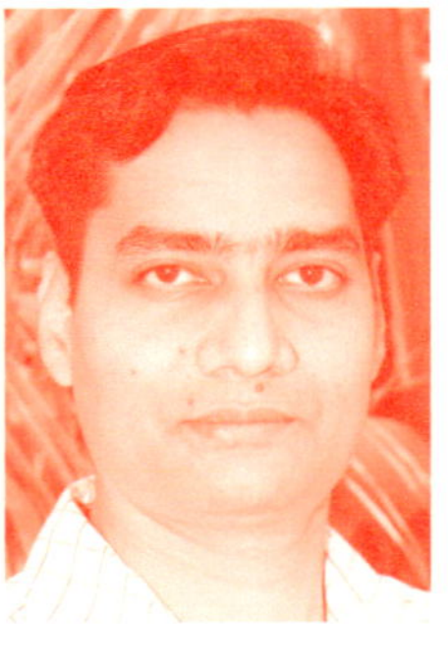
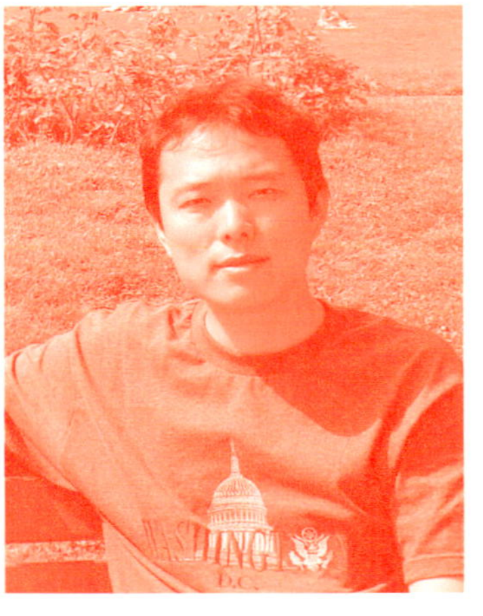
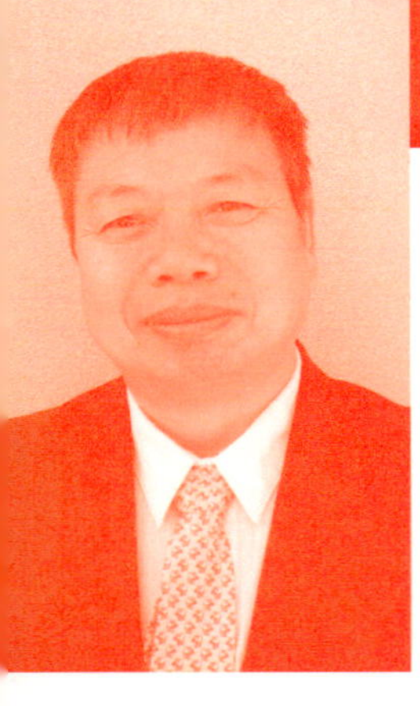
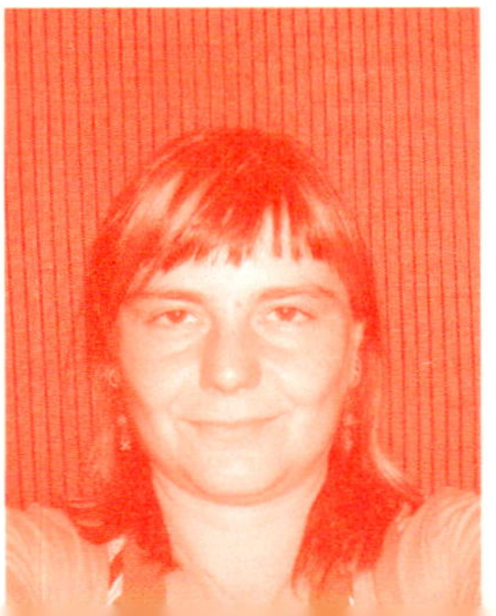

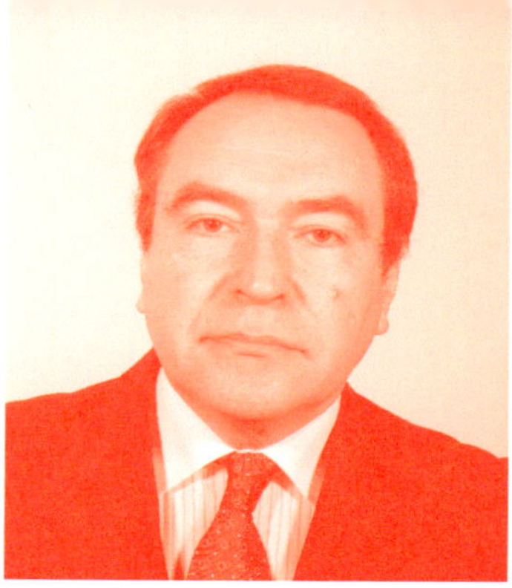
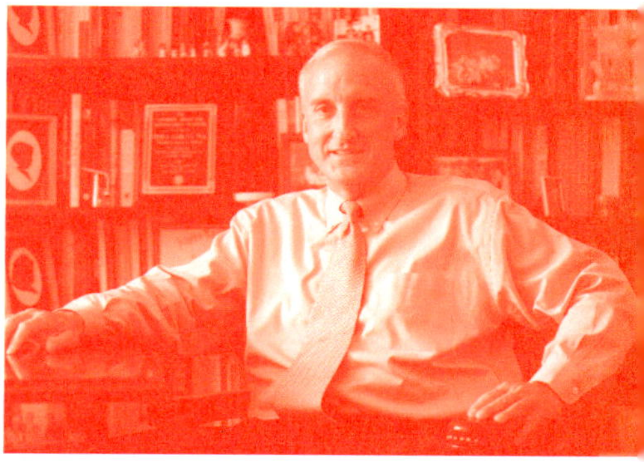
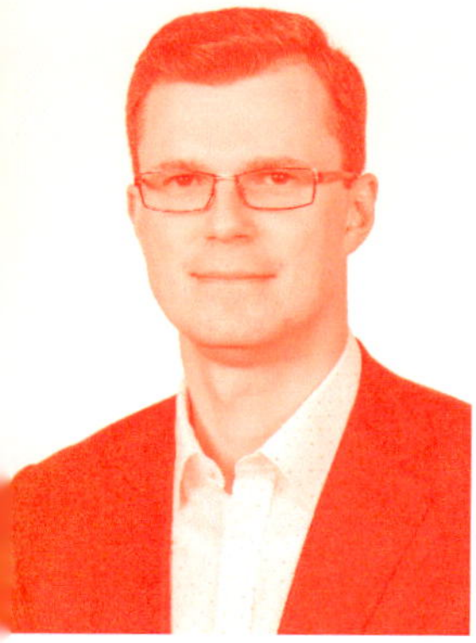
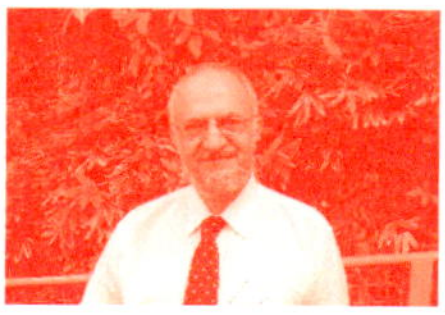
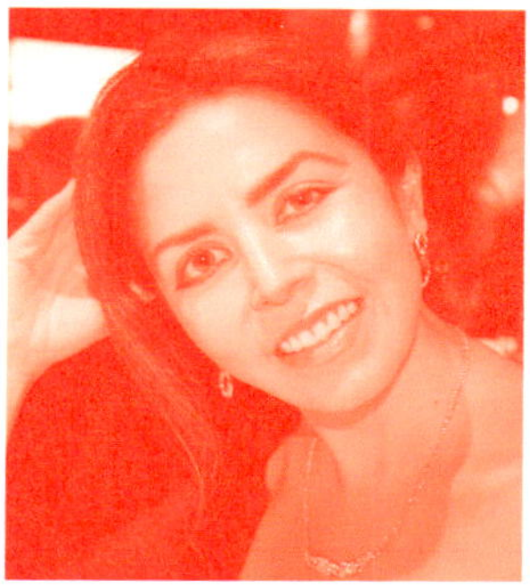

Supporting open minds since 2005

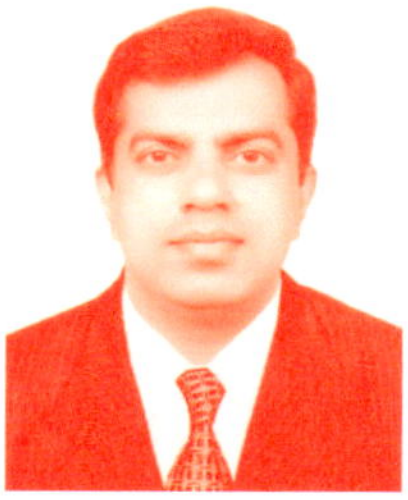
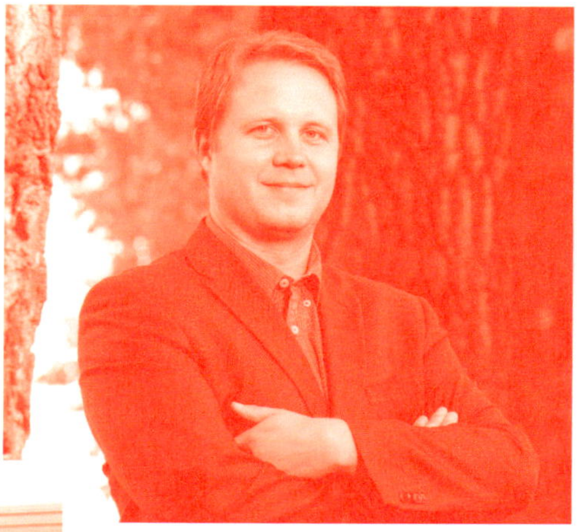
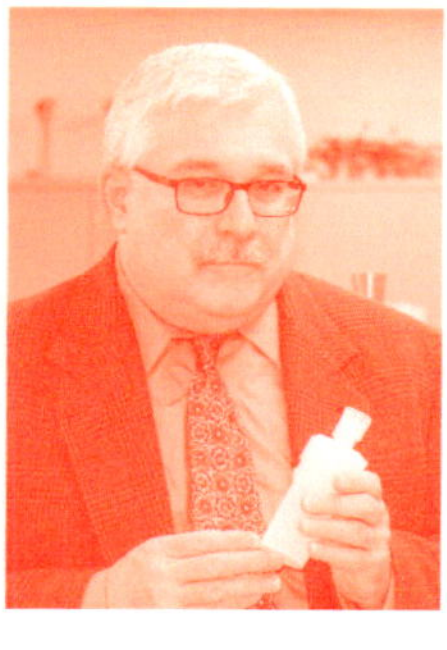
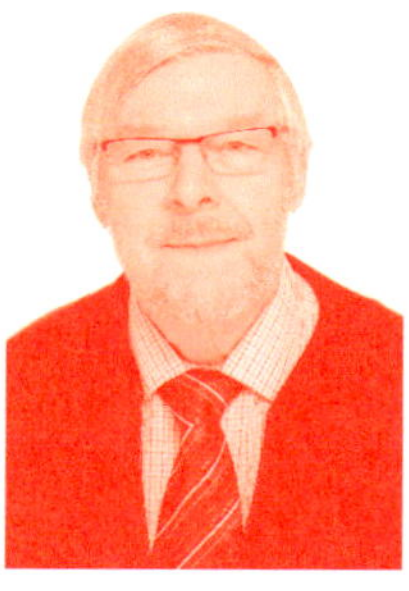
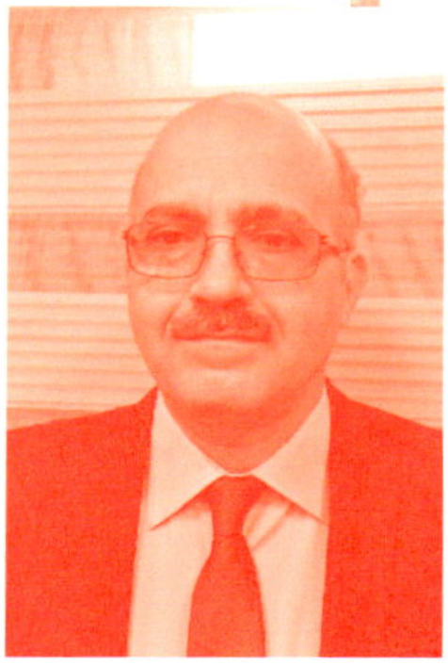
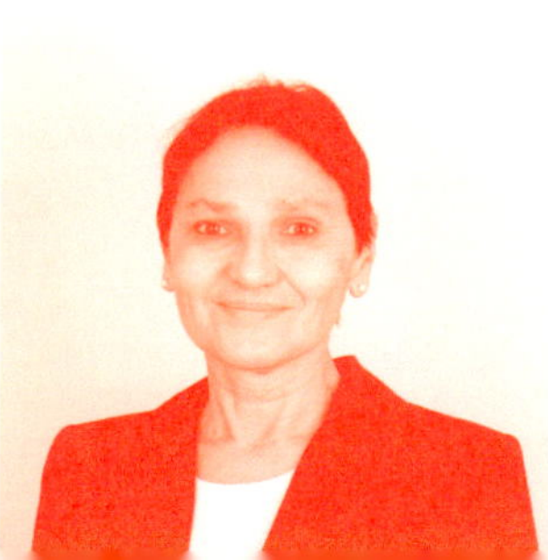
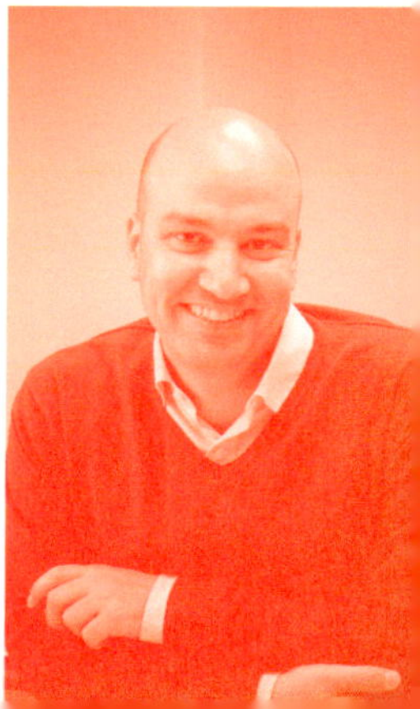

Advanced Studies in the 21st Century Animal Nutrition
http://dx.doi.org/10.5772/intechopen.92512
Edited by László Babinszky, Juliana Oliveira and Edson Mauro Santos

Part of IntechOpen Book Series: Veterinary Medicine and Science, Volume 8
Book Series Editor: Rita Payan-Carreira

Contributors
Tatien Masharabu, Joseph Butore, Jacques Nkengurutse, Mathias Hitimana, Daniel Sindaye, Sylvia I. Kehoe, Paweł Górka, Zhijun J. Cao, Douglas Nkosi, Meeske Robin, Sergio Alvarez, Ingrid Marumo Mokgadi Malebana, Francuois Muller, Cyprial Ncobela, Ronald S. Thomas, Magdalena Krauze, Jet Saartje Mandey, Florencia Nery Sompie, Halina Makała, Taşkın Değirmencioğlu, László Babinszky, Csaba Szabó, Márta Horváth, Arbab Sikandar

First published in London, United Kingdom, 2021 by IntechOpen
IntechOpen is the global imprint of INTECHOPEN LIMITED, registered in England and Wales, registration number: 11086078, 5 Princes Gate Court, London, SW7 2QJ, United Kingdom
Printed in Croatia

British Library Cataloguing-in-Publication Data
A catalogue record for this book is available from the British Library

Additional hard and PDF copies can be obtained from orders@intechopen.com

Advanced Studies in the 21st Century Animal Nutrition
Edited by László Babinszky, Juliana Oliveira and Edson Mauro Santos
p. cm.
Print ISBN 978-1-83969-403-5
Online ISBN 978-1-83969-404-2
eBook (PDF) ISBN 978-1-83969-405-9
ISSN 2632-0517

For EU product safety concerns:
IN TECH d.o.o., Prolaz Marije Krucifikse Kozulić 3, 51000 Rijeka, Croatia, info@intechopen.com or visit our website at intechopen.com.

IntechOpen Book Series

Veterinary Medicine and Science

Volume 8

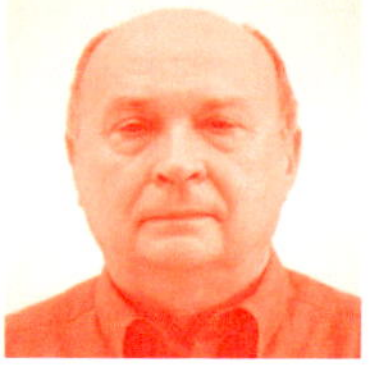

László Babinszky is Professor Emeritus, Department of Animal Nutrition Physiology, University of Debrecen, Hungary. He has also worked in the Department of Animal Nutrition, University of Wageningen, Netherlands; the Institute for Livestock Feeding and Nutrition (IVVO), Lelystad, Netherlands; the Agricultural University of Vienna (BOKU); the Institute for Animal Breeding and Nutrition, Austria; and the Oscar Kellner Research Institute for Animal Nutrition, Rostock, Germany. In 1992, Dr. Babinszky obtained a Ph.D. in Animal Nutrition from the University of Wageningen. His main research areas are swine and poultry nutrition. He has authored more than 300 publications (papers, book chapters) and edited four books and fourteen international conference proceedings.

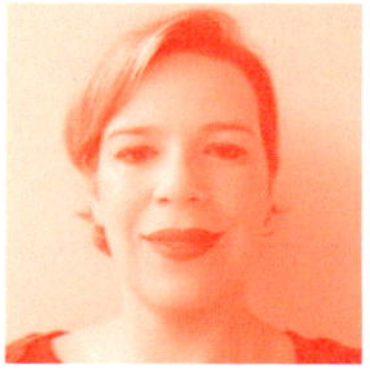

Juliana Oliveira is an associate professor at the Federal University of Paraíba (UFPB), Brazil, and a researcher for the Brazilian National Council for Scientific and Technological Development (CNPq). She obtained master's and doctoral degrees in Zootechnics from the Federal University of Viçosa (UFV), Brazil, in 2005 and 2008, respectively. Dr. Oliveira has been researching the use of forage in the diet of ruminant animals for more than twelve years.

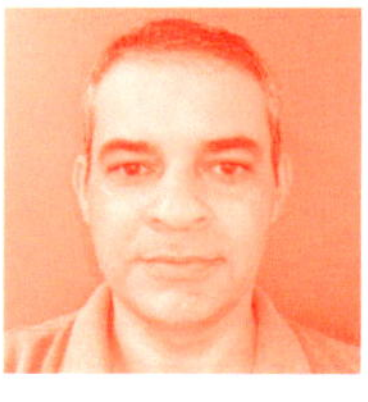

Dr. Santos is a Professor of Forage Crops and Pastures and Beef Cattle at the Federal University of Paraiba, Brazil. Dr. Santos received his Ph.D. in Animal Science (forage crops and ruminant nutrition) from the Federal University of Viçosa, Brazil, a master's degree in Animal Science, and a BS in Animal Science from the Federal Rural University of Rio de Janeiro (animal production). Dr. Santos' areas of interest include silage microbiology, cultivation and conservation of forage crops in semiarid regions, alternative feeds for ruminants, and pasture management. He is a researcher for INCT (National Institute of Science and Technology) - Animal Science, and a member of the Advisory Animal Science Committee of the Brazilian National Council for Scientific and Technological Development (CNPq).

Editors of Volume 8:
Prof. Dr. László Babinszky
University of Debrecen
Department of Animal Nutrition Physiology, Debrecen, Hungary

Dr. Juliana Oliveira
Dr. Edson Mauro Santos
Federal University of Paraíba, Federal University of Paraíba, Brazil

Book Series Editor: Rita Payan-Carreira
University of Évora, Portugal

Scope of the Series

Paralleling similar advances in the medical field, astounding advances occurred in the Veterinary Medicine and Science in recent decades, fostering a better support to animal health and more humane animal production, a better understanding of the physiology of endangered species, to improve the assisted reproductive technologies or the pathogenesis of certain diseases, where animals can be used as models for human diseases (like cancer, degenerative diseases or fertility), and even as a guarantee of public health. Bridging the Human, Animal and Environmental health, the holistic and integrative "One Health" concept intimately associates the developments within those fields, projecting its advancements into practice.
This book series aims to tackle a variety of fields in the animal-related medicine and sciences, providing thematic volumes, high quality and significance in the field, directed to researchers and postgraduates. It aims to give us a glimpse into the new accomplishments in the Veterinary Medicine and Science field. By addressing hot topics in veterinary sciences, we aim to gather authoritative texts within each issue of this series, providing in-depth overviews and analysis for graduates, academics and practitioners and foreseeing a deeper understanding of the subject. Forthcoming texts, written and edited by experienced researchers from both industry and academia, will also discuss scientific challenges faced today in Veterinary Medicine and Science. In brief, we hope that books in this series will provide accessible references for those interested or working in this field and encourage learning in a range of different topics.

Contents

Preface **XI**

Chapter 1 **1**
Impact of Selected Feed Additives in Broiler Nutrition on Breeding and the Meat Quality Features
by Halina Makała

Chapter 2 **19**
Phytogenic Feed Additives as An Alternative to Antibiotic Growth Promoters in Poultry Nutrition
by Jet Saartje Mandey and Florencia Nery Sompie

Chapter 3 **37**
Phytobiotics, a Natural Growth Promoter for Poultry
by Magdalena Krauze

Chapter 4 **59**
Use of *Bacillus Subtilis* Probiotics as Non-Antibiotic Gut Modulator and Growth Promoter in Broiler Chickens
by Arbab Sikandar

Chapter 5 **71**
Perspective Chapter: Using Feed Additives to Eliminate Harmful Effects of Heat Stress in Broiler Nutrition
by László Babinszky, Csaba Szabó and Márta Horváth

Chapter 6 **99**
Use of Aromatic Seeds as Feed Additives to Improve the Production of Anatolian Water Buffaloes
by Taşkın Değirmencioğlu

Chapter 7 **111**
Microbial Inoculation to High Moisture Plant By-Product Silage: A Review
by Bhutikini D. Nkosi, Cyprial N. Ncobela, Ronald S. Thomas, Ingrid M.M. Malebana, Francuois Müller, Sergio Álvarez and Robin Meeske

Chapter 8 **129**
Incorporating Silages into Preweaned Dairy Calf Diets
by Sylvia I. Kehoe, Paweł Górka and Zhijun J. Cao

Chapter 9 151
Bromatological Analysis of the Fodder Marketed in the Peri-Urban Areas of Bujumbura (Burundi): Towards Spontaneous Fodder Conservation by Transformation into Silage
by Joseph Butore, Daniel Sindaye, Mathias Hitimana, Jacques Nkengurutse and Tatien Masharabu

Preface

The field of animal nutrition aims to provide safe and high-quality foodstuffs as well as improve the efficiency of production and reduce environmental pollution. To achieve these goals, several serious challenges must be overcome.

The world's population is growing rapidly and there is an increasing demand for high-quality and safe food. At the same time, agricultural areas are diminishing due to industrialization, building of new motorways, new city construction programs, urbanization, and natural soil erosion. The fact that the Earth's climate has changed dramatically over the past decade is also increasing the pressure on agricultural production. Thus, under deteriorating environmental conditions, agriculture (including animal husbandry) needs to produce more and better foodstuffs, with less strain on our environment. More awareness and activity of participation is needed in animal production and nutrition to supply quality, environmentally friendly, and safe food in sufficient quantities. Therefore, the efficiency of animal production needs to be improved. This can be achieved by enhancing biological efficiency, technological efficiency, and economic efficiency.

It is well known that the efficiency of nutrition can be improved in several ways, including feeding animals with diets that meet their nutrient requirements, supplying nutrients according to age group and genetic profile, using good-quality and safe feed ingredients, using appropriate feed processing and additives, and so on.

Animal food additives are products used in animal nutrition for purposes of improving the quality of feed or the animal's performance and health. Other additives can be used to enhance digestibility or even flavor of feed materials. In addition, feed additives are known to improve the quality of compound feed production, thus improving the quality of a granulated mixed diet.

It is also a well-known fact that the quality of animal-origin foodstuffs can be improved by animal nutrition, but unfortunately, the reverse is also true. This finding is also valid for feed additives and feed processing (making silage).

This book focuses on some newer aspects of the various feed additives in poultry nutrition and of making silage in dairy cattle nutrition. It discusses the impact of the most important feed additives on broiler production and their mode of action in hot environments. It also demonstrates the use of plant-origin feed additives (aromatic seeds) in water buffalo nutrition, how to use silage in pre-weaned calf nutrition, and microbial inoculation in dairy cow nutrition.

Finally, the book examines the possibility of silage making for dairy cattle in peri-urban areas of developing countries.

This book is recommended for scientists, graduate students, and those working in the field of agriculture.

We would like to thank all the chapter authors for their excellent contributions. We are also grateful to the staff at IntechOpen, particularly Author Service Manager Maja Bozicevic and Commissioning Editor Lucija Tomicic-Dromgool.

Dr. László Babinszky
Professor,
Department of Animal Nutrition Physiology,
University of Debrecen,
Debrecen, Hungary

Dr. Juliana Oliveira and Dr. Edson Mauro Santos
Federal University of Paraíba,
Brazil

Chapter 1

Impact of Selected Feed Additives in Broiler Nutrition on Breeding and the Meat Quality Features

Halina Makała

Abstract

The aim of the study was to overview the results of scientific research on the impact of feed additives used in broiler nutrition on breeding and meat quality. Selected additives used in feeding broilers with immunomodulatory properties, prebiotics and probiotics, herbs and herbal extracts and protein additives were characterised. The application of insects in poultry feeding as a good source of proteins and fat as a substitute of expensive feed rich in proteins was presented. Further research is needed on their nutritional value, levels of incorporation into diets and the performance of this feed ingredient. However, there are many challenges that need to be overcome by adoptingsuitable strategies to produce antibiotic-free broiler meat with regards to food safety and chickenwelfare issues. The additives available on the market should be used in accordance with the manufacturers' recommendations and the grace period should be observed in order to obtain the expected production results and a high-quality product.

Keywords: feed additives, broiler nutrition, meat quality

1. Introduction

Commercial breeding programs are aimed at the maximisation of production results (rate of growth, fodder use, meat content, layer production), achievable in typical environmental conditions. The task of rational animal feeding is the achievement of a maximum production results but also keeping good state of health by favourable influence on gastrointestinal tract, metabolism and stimulation of immune system. It is especially important in feeding animals of a big production potential, including poultry.

In broiler nutrition special attention should be paid to additives of immuno-modulating action like: pre- and probiotics, yeast extracts, herbs and herb extracts.

The aim of the study was to overview the results of scientific research on the impact of feed additives used in broiler nutrition on breeding and meat quality.

2. About feed additives in general

Feed additives are the substances, microorganisms or preparations intentionally added to full-portion mixes and feeding doses in order to get improvement of their feeding usability: flavour, taste, consistency, dietetic values as well as extension of validity time (shelf-life). By applying them in animal feeding, including broilers, one can achieve higher daily growths, better fodder use, higher resistance to diseases, improvement of animal product quality and reduction of harmful effect of animal droppings on environment. In order to avoid improper dosage and uneven dispersion of an active substance in the mix, their application, both during production of mixes and direct feeding in farms should remain under constant control [1, 2]. Administration of functional feed additives, including direct-fed microorganisms (DFM), dietary prebiotics, and phytogenic preparations, has been demonstrated to improve growthperformance, animal health, and microbial food safety in poultry and is thought to be apotentially important component of antibiotic-free poultry production [3, 4].

Additives applicable to feed and water are an inherent feeding poultry component. Their application is connected with numerous advantages, but – at the same time – is subject to a strict control aimed mostly at avoidance of application not in accordance with their intended use. The classification, kind and scope of application of feed additives are regulated by the EU Law and regulations of Member States [5]. Additionally, consumer demand for antibiotic-free broiler meat is increasing. However, there are many challenges that need to be overcome by adopting suitable strategies to produce antibiotic-free broiler meat with regards to food safety and chicken welfare issues (**Table 1**) [6].

Following the withdrawal of antibiotic growth stimulators in poultry feeding, feed additives are applied, aimed at a favourable effect on bird's health and production parameters. The following additives are distinguished: those completing lacks of determined feeding components in the applied feed; supporting digestion processes; maintaining microbiological balance in gastrointestinal tract; improving productivity; reducing negative effect of droppings on natural environment; improving animal origin product quality; improving feeding value of feed additives; preventing diseases (in poultry production: coccidiosis and histomoniasis); facilitating production of feed mixes (binders, sticks). From the farmers' point of view the most important are the additives that have a direct influence on metabolism of the gastrointestinal tract of birds and regulate the level of provision in biologically active substances, since they increase production results. Among them we can include: vitamins and provitamins; mineral additives; amino acids, their salts and hydroxy analogues; digestion stimulators; stabilisers of intestinal microbiome; coccydiostatics [5]. While determining the dose of fodder and additives for hens and other poultry one should take into account their specie, body mass, age, production intensity, physiological state, gender, environment temperature and maintenance system [10].

The use and development of enzymes, phytogenics, prebiotics and probiotics has gained momentum in poultry feeding. The enzymes widely used by the industry are the non-starch polysaccharidases that cleave the non-starch polysaccharides in viscous cereals, microbial phytases that target the phytate-complexes in plant ingredients. Proteases are of interest to improve protein and amino acid digestibility, particularly in very young animals. Phytogenics are an alternative to in-feed antibiotics to prevent the risk of developing pathogens and also to satisfy consumer demand for a food chain free of drugs. Probiotic feed additives generally consist of one single strain or a combination of several strains of bacteria, *Bacillus spores* or yeasts species. Prebiotics are non-digestible food ingredients, such as fructo-oligosaccharides, xylooligo-saccharides, mannan-oligo-saccharides and galacto-oligosaccharides that are also used in feeds to protect poultry against pathogens [9].

Alternatives to antibiotics	Active ingredients	Basic functions	Effects on broiler
Probiotics	*Bacillus subtilis, Enterococcus faecium Lactobacillus acidophilus, Bacilluslicheniformis, Bifidobacterium bifidum*	Appetite anddigestion, stimulant, antioxidant	Increased body weight and FCR Improved absorptive surface of duodenum andileum Increase nutrient retention
Prebiotics	Fructo-oligosaccharides (FOS), inulin, galacto-oligosaccharides (GOS), trans-galacto oligosaccharides	Digestion, stimulant	Increased growth performance Stimulation of metabolic activity in intestine
Organic acids	Citric acid Ascorbic acid Propionic acid and sodium bentonite Butyrate	Digestion, stimulant, increased feed effciency	Increased body weight Improved ileal nutrient digestibility, cell proliferation, and epithelial and villi height
Amino acids and enzymes	Phytase, lysins	Digestion, stimulant	Improved growth performance
Phytogenic feed additives	Pepper	Digestion, stymulant	No effect on live performance
	Garlic	Digestion,stimulant, Antiseptic	Higher body weight
	Ginger	Gastric stymulant	No effects on performance
	Rosemary	Digestion, stimulant, antiseptic, antioxidant	Improved live weight and feed effciency
	Thyme		No significant effect on BW/FCR
	Mint	Appetite, digestion, stimulant, antiseptic	Decreased serum total cholesterol, triglycerides, and low-density lipoprotein concentration
Nanoparticles (NPs)	Silver NPs Selenium NPs Copper NPs Metal NPs such as zinc oxide, zirconium dioxide, and platinum Zn-bearing zeolite clinoptilolite NPs Nanosuspensions of clay minerals	Digestion, Stimulant	Increased body weight and FCR

Source: [4, 6–9].

Table 1.
Alternatives to antibiotics and their functions and impacts on broiler production.

3. Additives of immunomodulating action applicable in broiler feeding

Contagious diseases, in spite of ever improving prevention programs, cause big losses in poultry production, and foodstuffs contaminated with pathogens may be dangerous for consumers. In order to increase poultry resistance against pathogenic factors, more and more additives of immunomodulating character are applied in fodder industry. The effect of immunomodulators consists in their direct action on the cells of the immune system that ensure an immune response. Modification of the process of determined immune reactions in this way increases the organism resistance to viral, bacterial and parasite infections. The immuno-modulating feed additives include: pre- and probiotics, components of baker's yeast cell walls (mannooligosaccharides, ß-glucan and nucleotides) and herbal extracts (echinacea, aloe and ginseng). Certain amino acids (arginine, methionine), vitamins (E, A, C), microelements (Zn, Sn) and fatty acids (LC PUFA n-3, CLA) also play an important role in the immune processes in poultry [5, 11].

The withdrawal of antibiotic growth stimulators resulted in increased interest in immunomodulators that stimulate GALT. These are, among others, prebiotics. They are applicable in fodder industry in order to increase poultry resistance to pathogenic factor action [12, 13]. Recently, interest in probiotics and prebiotics as feed additives that may constitute an important factor inhibiting multiplication of intestinal pathogens at poultry fed with mixes non containing antibiotic growth stimulators has increased [14]. Immunostimulating action of this kind of feed additives is also an important issue.

Lipiński and others [12] examined the effect of application of a prebiotic preparation containing mannanoligosaccharides in mixes for broiler chicken, for their health status and meat quality. In fodder mixes, instead of a plant stimulator and acidifier (control group), the prebiotic preparation Biolex MB 40 (mannanoligosaccharides) was applied in the quantity of 2 kg/t of mix (group II). In the experimental group III the preparation Biolex MB 40 in the quantity of 2 kg/t and acidifier were applied. In result of studies at chicken fed with mixes with the participation of the tested preparation, the activation of non-specific defence mechanism against infection was noted, proved by the increase of the level of lysozyme in blood serum. The meat of the test chicken was characterised by a similar content of dry mass, raw ash, total protein and raw fat. The application of the tested preparation at the chicken for slaughter had no influence on the chemical composition of meat (**Table 2**).

Vidanarachchi et al. [15] examined the effect of action of two different extracts of carbohydrates soluble in water (extract from renga renga lily and acacia) and two prebiotic compounds available in the market, Fibregum and Raftifeed-IPE, on productivity of broiler chicken subject to the provocation of necrotic (necrotising)

Item	Control	Biolex MB 40	Biolex MB 40 + acidifier	SEM
Lysozyme [mg/l]	6,84a	7,99b	9,14c	0,261
Dry matter [%]	26,24	25,90	25,92	0,105
Ash [%]	1,20	1,18	1,18	0,013
Protein [%]	22,30	22,07	21,96	0,079
Fat [%]	2,92	3,01	2,86	0,085

a, b – different letters in a row differ significantly $p \leq 0.05$.
Source: [14].

Table 2.
Level of lysozyme in blood serum of broiler chickens and chemical composition of breast meat.

enteritis (NE). These therapies were compared to the negative and positive controls (bacitracin Zn). Total 8,8% death rate connected with NE was noted, with the average assessment of changes in jejunum and ileum at dead birds in the range of 3,03 to 3,90 at all provoked groups except for positive control groups. Neither specific deaths for NE nor clinical irregularities with unquestioned control groups and positive control groups were noted. In result of the studies it has been proved that supplementation with carbohydrates soluble in water from two plant (herbal) sources was not effective against NE controlling. It has been proved, however, that the prebiotic compound Fibregum has certain immunomodulating action. Addition of bacitracin Zn and monensins was highly effective in counteracting negative effects of the disease.

4. Pre- and probiotics applicable in poultry feeding

Prebiotics are the substances that have to fulfil certain requirements. They must not be digested in upper sections of the gastrointestinal tracts, they should stimulate development of a favourable intestinal microbiome, and products of their decomposition should lower pH of the digestive tract content. Prebiotics are substrates selectively and in a better way utilised by bifidobacteria and other species of favourable bacteria, and mainly fermentation products of these compounds. Short-chain fatty acids lower pH of intestinal environment and worsen conditions of development of bacteria undesirable in poultry breeding (*Clostridium, Salmonella*). The bioactive substances in the form of prebiotics, most frequently applicable to birds, comprise fructooligosaccharides, inulin obtained from chicory roots, oligofructose and manno oligosaccharides. Moreover, one can meet isomaltooligosaccharides, soya oligosaccharides, galaktooligosacharydy, maltooligosaccharides, glucooligosaccharides and xylooligo-saccharides [5]. Probiotics can replace antibiotics by changing the intestinal microbiome, thereby producing some of the effects of antibiotics. For example, feed supplementation with probiotics improves the feed effciency and intestinal health and, ultimately, facilitates the faster growth of broilers by reducing the intestinal pH, altering the intestinal bacterial composition, and improving digestive activity. Probiotics stimulate endogenous enzyme production, which reduces the production of toxic substances and increases vitamins and/or antimicrobials such as bacteriocins [6].

Probiotics are the preparations containing desired intestinal microflora, among others *Lactobacillus acidophilus, L. bulgaricus, L. casei, L. reuterii, Bifidobacterium bifidum, B. longum* and others. Administered in the form of live bacteria or endospores they have a favourable effect on host health improving intestinal microbiological balance. The mechanism of activity of probiotics is multiway and it consists, among others, in: restoring and maintaining natural balance of gastrointestinal tract microflora; protection of gastrointestinal tract against pathogens; production of bacteriocins, short-chain organic acids; synthesis of vitamins of group B, vitamin K and digestion enzymes; stimulation of immune system; reduction of concentration of toxic substances in gastrointestinal tract and in blood; lowering pH of intestinal content, cholesterol and triglycerides level in blood and tissues [5].

Broiler feed supplemented with *B. subtilis* increased the body weights by 4.4%. The H_2S and NH_3 concentrations in chicken excretions were also reduced after treating chickens with probiotics, leading to less odour. Probiotics increased the meat quality of poultry by affecting the fat and protein contents [6].

Mixed feed additives called synbiotics (preparation containing pre- and probiotics at the same time) are also worth consideration, containing in their composition lactic acid bacteria of the species *Lactobacillus, Bacillus*, *Bifidoacterium and Enterococcus* [8].

Immunomodulating action of pre-, pro- and synbiotics is connected with the action of lactic acid bacilli in the organism. It is manifested, first of all, by favourable influence on development and activities of immune system at the level of intestinal mucosa (GALT). Feed additives with an immunomodulating effect constitute a valuable supplement compound feed for poultry. Their influence is based on the direct stimulation of the cells of the immune system, which increases the efficiency of the processes immunological and leads to lower susceptibility of birds to pathogenic microorganisms [11].

In studies on poultry it has been proved that chicken for slaughter, given probiotic preparation containing *Lactobacillus acidophilus, Bifidobacterium bifidum* and *Streptococcus faecalis* characterise, as compared to the control group, with higher immunoglobulin level (especially IgM) in blood serum directed against SRBC antigen, but there was no effect of probiotic in response to BSA antigen [11, 16].

At chicken for layers the preparation containing live *Lactobacillus casei* strains had a positive effect for humoral mechanisms of resistance, substantially increasing production of antibodies after immunisation with virus of supposed poultry pest or with BSA antigen [11, 17].

Broiler chicken Ross 308 fed with diets with addition of symbiotic containing bacteria *Bacillus subtilis* C-3102 and yeast (*Saccharomyces cerevisiae*) in the ratio 1:1 were characterised with higher slaughter productivity. The birds were reared for 42 days. Chickens were given *ad libitum*, wheat-corn-soybean mixtures and wheat-triticale-soybean. Application of fodder additive, irrespective of the kind of grain in mixes resulted in the lowering of the mass of the chicken gastrointestinal tract and increase of the mass of edible giblets. It has been proved that the combination of probiotic and prebiotic bacteria may be a good fodder additive stimulating growth and development of broiler chicken. However, while choosing a given preparation one should take into account many factors, mainly quality and specificity of the preparation, direction of production and kind of diet [8].

The increasing interest in probiotics and herbal additives in poultry feeding results from their favourable influence of health state of the gastrointestinal tract and reduction of intestinal problems. In many research programs a favourable influence of additives stabilising gastrointestinal tract microbiome on poultry production results was proved [18]. The influence of probiotics on production results is less stable than that of herbal additives. Certain researches proved minor influence of probiotics on

Specification	**Control**	***Lactobacillus lactis***	**Essential oil**
Duration of trial (days)	105	105	105
Final body weight (g)	9,03B	9,32A	9,11B
FCR (kg/kg)	2,34	2,36	2,31
Mortality rate (%)	96,25	96,25	96,25
EEI* (pts)	353,4	362,7	361,6
Dry matter (%)	26,72	26,52	26,46
Ash (%)	1,20	1,19	1,20
Protein (%)	25,76	25,36	25,64
Fat (%)	0,41	0,38	0,48

A, B – different letters in a row differ significantly $p \leq 0.05$.
Source: [19].

Table 3.
Productivity results of the turkeys during the trial period and chemical composition of breast meat.

productivity but the majority of them confirm at least favourable trends in production results, equalisation of animals, lowering death and incidence ratio or lowering of treatment costs after application of probiotics in fodder [19, 20].

Results of research works of Lipiński and others [19] on influence of probiotic and herbal additives on productivity and quality of turkey meat proved that application of a probiotic preparation in mixes for turkeys for slaughter resulted in improvement of production results expressed in body mass but had no influence on use of fodder and health of birds. Application of a herbal preparation in mixes for turkeys had no influence on fattening. The meat of test turkeys was characterised with a similar content of dry mass, raw ash, total protein and raw fat (**Table 3**). The analysis of the European efficiency ratio showed that the use of the tested feed additives had a positive effect on the value of this indicator. The best results in this respect were found in birds from group II (362.7 vs. 353.4 in the control group) and III (361.6 vs. 353.4 in the control group); however, the differences found were not statistically significant [19].

5. Herbs and herb extracts

Modern methods of poultry breeding are aimed at elimination or reduction of use of chemical means in animal feeding. One of the ways towards that end is the return to use natural fodder additives, like herbs. Herb fodder additives are at present of growing interest in connection with total prohibition of use of antibiotics.

Herbs and herbal (phytogenic) additives in animal feeding act favourably on increase of animal resistance and reduction of incidence ratio, improving animal welfare. Herbs do not add nutrition substances but they improve taste and digestibility of fodder thus increasing its use. The research enabling identification of active substances in herbs and determination of their action on the organism resulted in their more rational application and better adjustment to the needs. Herbs contain various kinds of active substances like essential oils, dyestuffs, alkaloids, glycosides, phenolic acids, phytosterols, flavonoids. Activity of active substances contained in herbs and medicinal plants is usually multi way. Their action is immuno-stimulating, anti-inflammatory, antibacterial and they improve quality of products of animal origin. They activate secretion of digestive juices, increase appetite and peristaltic of intestines as well as improve processes of absorption of nutritive components (**Table 4**) [5, 26].

Genre / production group	The form of feeding herbs			
	fresh	dried	dried extracts	oils
broilers	0	++	++	++
laying hen	+	++	+	++
gooses	++	0	0	0
turkeys	++	++	+	++
ducks	+	0	0	0

"+" - low efficiency (0-2% improvement);
"++" - desired effectiveness (2.1-5%);
"+++" - high efficiency (over 5%);
"0" - lack of effectiveness or information in the available literature.
Source: [7, 21–25].

Table 4.
Effectiveness of using herbs in animal nutrition.

The compounds of plant origin, the so-called phytobiotics, are also applicable in animal feeding in order to improve productivity and quality of products of animal origin. They are considered as natural and safe additives and their multi way action gives possibility of their wide use in animal feeding [27]. Particularly effective immunomodulating additives include phytogenic preparations (Echinacea, Aloe and Ginseng) [11].

The effectiveness of herbs applied in their natural forms may differ according to the time of harvesting, habitat conditions they grew in, conditions of drying and storage, and thus more and more herbal-mineral-aromatic preparations appear in the market. These are preparations like BioStrong, Dominal as well as Digestarom, containing essential oils of peppermint, marjoram, cloves, anise and dill on an inorganic carrier [28].

Many research works confirm favourable influence of herbs on health of birds. The use of herbs in animal nutrition results not only from the taste preferences of animals, but also due to their influence on the organisms of animals - most often they have a therapeutic effect. Knowing the chemical composition and the effect of individual substances on the animal's body makes it possible to use herbs more rationally. Plants or parts of plants contain many different substances that actively interact with the animal's organism. The action of active substances in herbs and medicinal plants is most often multidirectional. They stimulate the secretion of digestive juices, increase appetite and intestinal peristalsis, and improve the absorption of nutrients. The advantage is also a positive effect on the body through anti-diarrheal, anti-inflammatory, antiparasitic and antipyretic properties [5].

Biologically active substances contained in herbs like essential oils, tannins, glycosides, flavonoids, terpen, mucus, organic acids show various actions: antibacterial [29], antiviral, antimycotic, immunostimulating [30] and antistress [24]. Many active substances contained in herbs improve taste and flavour values of products of animal origin, and first of all discolour egg yolks, as well as bond mycotoxins [5]. In poultry prophylaxis and treatment herbs may be used as entire plants or their particular parts only: in a fresh and dried form, in the form of infusions, brews, essences, extracts, macerates and essential oils [25].

Arczewska-Włosek and Świątkiewicz [31] inform that thanks to the properly selected herb extracts added to the fodder mix there is a possibility of replacing coccydiostatics. It has been proved that the mix of sage extracts (*Salvia officinalis*), garlic (*Allium sativum*), purple echinacea (*Echinacea purpurea*), thyme (*Thymus vulgaris*) and oregano (*Origanum vulgare*) had a positive influence on production results of birds infected with oocysts *Eimeria* sp.. According to Majewska et al. [32], herbs introduced to poultry diet may lower cholesterol concentration in blood and thus affect positively birds' health. Hipocholesterolemic effect results from the fact that chemical compounds contained in plant essential oils, e.g. citral, geraniol, cineol, menton, menthol, fenchon, borneol, fenchyl, may cause inhibition of liver enzyme activity (reductase HMGCoA), that controls quantity of synthetised cholesterol and thus lowers its concentration in blood [24, 33].

Phytogenic feed additives may also improve fodder taste and thus increase its intake and improve production results, including fodder consumption and use and growth of poultry body mass [27]. Unambiguous confirmation of the positive effect of herbs on production results of broiler chicken is still problematic, since obtained results are often contradictory. Kwiecień et al. [22] and Kwiecień and Winiarska-Mieczan [23] proved positive influence of herbs on hen broiler body mass but Brzóska et al. [7] and Gardzielewska et al. [28] drew different conclusions. Gardzielewska et al. [28] examined influence of application of Digestarom preparation and charcoal on quality of fresh meat and after 4-month storage frozen. Tests were conducted on broiler cocks Ross 308. In result of the tests it has been proved that Digestarom preparation resulted in brightening of muscle colour, substantially bigger acidification, increasing of losses of meat juice both during defreezing and cooking, worsening of sensorial properties of meat and bullion, as well and increase of cholesterol level. It was also proved that the addition of Digestarom preparation affected adversely the majority of tested meat properties after defreezing and cooking. However, the addition of charcoal affected positively the reduction of meat losses after storage and cooking and sensorial assessment of cooked meat and bullion.

Adequate feeding of broiler chicken may, to a certain extent, control fat content in meat and modify its composition leading to the product of desired nutrition and dietetic features. Phytogenic fodder compounds, including resin *Boswellia serrata* are helpful in this matter. In the tests conducted by Kiczorowska et al. [34] it has been proved that the application of Boswellia resin in feeding broilers decreased content of C14 and C18:3 acids and increased total KTJN in the fat of breast muscles. However, its use in ecologic fodders resulted in increasing quantity of C18:3 acid in the fat of chicken breast muscles.

Broiler chicken show lower resistance to environmental factors and higher sensibility to stress states what affects negatively their productivity and health [35]. At present growing attention is paid to the possibilities of using herbs in counteracting stress situations during breeding.

From many plants of immunomodulating activities the best known are certain species of echinacea (*Echinacea purpurea*, *E. angustifolia*, *E. pallida*). They come from The North America where they have been applicable as medicinal herbs for ages. The immuno-stimulating property of echinacea covers various kinds of resistance and it is a representative of actions of many substances contained in this plant, i.e. coffee acid derivatives (coffee acid, quornic acid, echinakozide, verbassoside and others), non-starch polysaccharides (heteroxylans, arabinoramnogalactans), alkaloids (mainly isobuthyloamides) and essential oils and flavonoids. Immunomodulating properties of echinacea were duly documented in clinical tests on human and in model tests on rats and mice [11].

Ginseng (*Panax ginseng*) contains active substances of actions stimulating phagocyte activity of macrophages, activity of NK cells, production of relay cytokines and IgM and other immunoglobulins, as well as T lymphocyte proliferation. In experiments with chicken for slaughter infected with Salmonella gallinarum bacteria, application of a preparation with ginseng in drinking water reduced rate of death, extent of liver infection and number of birds in droppings of which cultures of tested bacteria were found [11, 36].

In tests on turkey hens for slaughter a preparation containing active substance of aloe, chokeberry and vitamin C increased total quantity of leucocytes and activity of lysozyme in blood, and phagocyte activity of leucocytes against *Staphylococcus aureus* bacteria. At chicken infected with *Salmonella gallinarun* bacteria or virus of supposed poultry pest the addition of aloe reduced rate of death and increased synthesis of IL-6 [11, 37].

6. Protein rich feed additives

Fodder quality and especially quantity and quality of proteins contained therein are of a basic importance in animal feeding. Protein is a component necessary for proper growth and functioning of an animal organism. Its use is optimum if the amino acid composition and mutual proportions of amino acids correspond to the needs that depend on production group, gender, age and body mass of animals [10].

In feeding hens the grain corns are basic being the main source of energy. Grain may constitute 40 to 80% of the dose. Not all grains, however, are recommended. In the poultry diet the first amino acid limiting growth is methionine together with cystine. The majority of raw fodders is of a big shortage of methionine. It is an important problem for farmers since thanks to methionine the animal organisms are able to produce creatine, choline or epinephrine. Each excess of amino acids is eliminated from the organism in the form of ammonia, and that is why it is so important that the supplied proteins were of full value. Loss of this valuable component results in production cost growth and increases environmental contamination in result of emission of nitrogen to soil, ground waters and air [10].

Rich chemical composition of lucerne concentrate, high content of proteins, amino acids, dyes, vitamins, mineral components, energy and other active substances results in its application in animal feeding as plant fodder additive (phytobiotic) instead of the withdrawn antibiotic growth stimulators [38, 39]. Biologically active compounds contained in lucerne concentrate support immune and haematopoietic system of fed animals [38, 40]. In tests with feed additive Polisavone, extract from lucerne, it has been proved that it increased resistance and lowered the content of lard fat at chicken but did not increase body mass growth and fodder use by these birds [40]. The studies of Ognik and Czech [41] have proved that the addition of lucerne concentrate (PX) to turkey diet resulted in a total growth of antioxidation capacity and growth of vitamin C and copper in blood of these birds.

Goronowicz et al. [42] assessed selected physical and chemical features of breast muscles of chicken for slaughter from ecologic and intensive breeding. Compound feed with additives for chicken of ecologic breeding was prepared according to the criteria, it was poorer as regards basic nutrition components. It contained less proteins and metabolic energy. In result of tests it was proved that muscles of chicken for slaughter of ecologic breeding were characterised with good nutrition value (more proteins, less fat) and they were of a darker colour, what may be a desirable feature for many consumers. However, high pH_{24} of breast muscles of chicken of ecologic breeding indicates that their meat may be vulnerable to microbiological infections and may be stored for a short time only. Moreover, it needs more force for cutting what may indicate that it has to be subject to a longer thermal processing.

Algae may be an interesting protein additive in poultry feeding. Algae may be obtained from natural sources or cultivated in artificial ponds, e.g. phototrophic microalgae. The most popular alga is spirulina, used in many countries as an additive to food for people and animals due to its big nutrition value. Spirulina (*Arthrospira platensis*) belongs to unicellular microalgae living in natural or artificial water reservoirs. Tests proved that adding microalgae to fodder in poultry feeding increase content of unsaturated fatty acids (NNKT) and carotenoids in egg yolks. The best results were noted in a group of 10% additive of algae in which the biggest growth of body mass, decrease of fat content in blood and liver were noted, as compared to control group [21].

7. New generation of protein rich feed additives (insect and fly protein)

The poultry production market is expected to grow constantly and dynamically. This fact results from, among others, high nutritive value of products (meat, eggs), their relatively low price and lack of consumption contraindications resulting from religious limitations. Moreover, in the time of global warming, poultry is characterised with a relatively low emission of greenhouse gases, as compared to other farm animals. However, intensification of poultry production needs increasing supply of various protein sources in the diet [43].

Recently, the use of various species of insects as the source of protein and fat in poultry feeding has been noted. In many countries, including Asia, Africa and Latin America, invertebrates constitute common source of protein in fodder mixes for farm animals [44]. Nutrition specialists, looking for new unique protein sources to be used in broiler feeding, conduct studies on influence of share of flours (meal) made of insect larvae on productivity of chicken for slaughter and on development of microbiome in their intestines [45]. Józefiak and others [45] consider insects as a valuable alternative source of proteins and fat in poultry feeding, as a substitute of expensive fodders rich in proteins. Insects may supplement fodders like soya, maize (corn), cereals or fish meal. The production of meal (flour) from insects is ecologic because it does not use water; it is characterised with low emission of greenhouse gases and processing of raw materials of low value into valuable proteins. The chemical composition of various species of insects is highly differentiated and thus it needs standardisation of production processes of meal that, added to broiler fodders, has no influence on breeding results significantly modifying microflora of their gastrointestinal tracts [45, 46]. The concentration of nutrients in the meal supplemented with insects depends on their developmental stage, production conditions and composition of feed and substrates on which they are grown. Insects can play the Essentials role in animal nutrition, therefore studies on their nutritional value are required [2].

The composition of meals made from insects depends on insect species, their development stadium, production conditions, fodder composition and components of substrate they were bred on. Protein content in meal made from insects varies from 40–60%. Insect protein characterises with high digestibility (ca 85%) and its amino acid composition is more favourable than that of cereal proteins. Insect larvae contain also more fat than cereals or leguminous plants and thus they form a good source of energy. This fat is highly digestible and has a favourable profile of fatty acids (**Table 5**) [47].

Item	*Gryllus assimilis*		*Musca domestica)*		*Hermetia illucens*	*Tenebrio molitor*	*Blatta lateralis*
	Imago	**subimago**	**pupae**	**larvae**	**larvae**	**larvae**	**nymph**
Per kg DM							
Gross energy [MJ]	21.5	19.3	20.1	20.24	22.1	26.8-27.3	—
Crude fibre [g]	70	94	157	16-86	70	51-88	85-89
ash [g]	64	54	55-98	31-173	146-284	10-45	45-54
Phosphorus[g]	8.0	8.6	—	9.2-24.0	6.4-15.0	4.4-14.2	0.6-0.7
Calcium [g]	9.9	3.1	—	3.1-8.0	50.0-86.0	0.3-6.2	0.2
Crude protein [g]	564	638	630-762	380-604	411-450	451-603	543-734
Crude fat [g]	238	168	144-161	90-260	150-350	250-431	176-261
Fatty aids per kg fat							
SFAs [g]	351	352	476	417	749	229-334	28.7
MUFAs [g]	298	261	307	314	155	407-536	46.3-50.2
PU As [g]	336	369	291	399	74	254-323	138-219
Total PUFA *n-3* [g]	22	17	—	—	2	2-4	1-11
Total PUFA *n-6* [g]	314	352	—	—	23	81-93	35-207

Source: [2, 43–45].

Table 5.
Nutrient composition of different insect meals.

In tests on feeding of chicken for slaughter the test results concerning use of larvae of domestic flies are available. Test results show that addition of these insects in a mix may reach up to 25% without unfavourable effect on growth of body mass, fodder consumption and fodder use coefficient. High digestibility of amino acids was noted, in 95% at turkeys and in 91% at chicken for slaughter fed with meal from domestic fly larvae [43].

Insects' capacity of synthetising of anti-microorganism peptides encourages to use them in feeding of farm animals. High level of biocidal peptides (defensins) may play potential role of improvement of health and animal welfare. Józefiak and others [45] proved that a relatively small addition of *Shelfordella lateralis* (up to 0,2%) of peptides dried in low temperature (50°C) improved growth of body mass of chicken for slaughter. The obtained results suggest that addition of these insects may have influence on numerical amount of chicken intestinal microflora population and thus act anti-bacterially.

The published results concerning application of insect meal show that insects have a big potential in animal feeding. As a protein source they have an adequate amino acid profile. Histidine, lysine and tryptophan are limiting amino acids that may be included in the diet. Moreover, it is necessary to make assessment of profiles of amino acids of other insect species in order to select species of the best amino acid profile or improve the profile using genetic methods.
In order to introduce insects as fodder component in the food chain (fodder chain) additional studies concerning their nutritive value, level of introduction in diets and functional properties of this kind of fodder ingredient are necessary [2, 48].

At present an insufficient supply of insects, i.e. lack of professional high productivity farms as well as impossibility of guaranteeing constant deliveries, is an important barrier in the use of insect meals in animal feeding. Lack of technologies dedicated to insect production results in the cost of production being at present too high to compete with the currently used protein sources. However, the works on implementation of new fodder materials, i.e. insect meals in full proportions for farm animals including poultry are on the way and their expectations are promising [43, 48]. There are also concerns about the safety of the food that uses insect meal for animal nutrition. It is currently unclear whether insect protein contains viruses or prions. Some researchers are not sure if any heat treatment can neutralise these factors. Virologists are also not of the same opinion on this point. Therefore, further research is needed in this area.

8. Main conclusions

1. The use of feed additives to improve the efficiency of growth and/or eggs production, prevent disease and improve feed utilisation is a strategy to improve the efficiency of the poultry industry.

2. The use of feed additives in poultry production is inevitable and results from breeding progress, shortening the time of breeding, resulting in increased susceptibility of birds to environmental and nutritional conditions.

3. The additives available on the market should be used in accordance with the manufacturers' recommendations and the grace period should be observed in order to obtain the expected production results and a high-quality product.

4. The feed additives with immunomodulatory properties constitute a valuable supplement to the feed mixtures for poultry.

5. Promising results relate to the use and implementation of insect meal for poultry. Further research is needed on their nutritional value, levels of incorporation into diets and the performance of this feed ingredient.

8.1 Suggestions for practice

1. The growing global demand for poultry meat and changes in consumer preferences as regards the quality of poultry products have an impact on the modification of feeding methods and composition of poultry feed mixtures.

2. Adopting appropriate strategies for the production of broiler meat without antibiotics presents challenges in terms of food safety and chicken welfare.

Author details

Halina Makała
Division of Meat and Fat Technology, Institute of Agricultural and Food Biotechnology - State Research Institute, Warsaw, Poland

*Address all correspondence to: halina.makala@ibprs.pl

References

[1] Szostak B. 2015. Dodatki paszowe stosowane w żywieniu świń. „Trouw i MY" 3(39) : 12-14.

[2] Weiner A., Paprocka I., Kwiatek K. 2018. Wybrane gatunki owadów jako źródło składników odżywczych w paszach. Życie Weterynaryjne, 93(7) : 499-504.

[3] Broderick T. J.,Gutierrez O.,† Lee J. T., Duong T. 2021. Evaluation of functional feed additive administrationin broiler chickens to 21 d. Journal of Applied Poultry Research. Volume 30, Issue 2, June 2021, 100121 : 1-13.

[4] Mehdi Y., Letourneau-Montminy M.P., Gaucher M.L., Chorfi Y., Suresh G., Rouissi T., Brar S.K., Cot C., Ramirez A.A., Godbout S. 2018. Use of antibiotics in broiler production: Global impacts and alternatives. Animal Nutrition. 4 (2018) : 170-178.

[5] Mituniewicz T. 2015. Dodatki paszowe dla drobiu. Agri Food, OID, (283)4 : 20-27.

[6] Haque H., Sarker S., Islam S., Islam A., Karim R., Hoque Kayesh M.E., Muhammad Shiddiky J. A., Anwer M. S. 2020. Sustainable Antibiotic-Free Broiler Meat Production: Current Trends, Challenges, and Possibilities in a Developing Country Perspective. Biology. 2020, 9, 0411 : 1-24.

[7] Brzóska F., Śliwiński B., Michalik-Rutkowska O. 2010. Effect of herb mixture on productivity, mortality, carcass quality and blond parameters of broiler chickens. Annals of Animal Science, 10(2) : 157-165.

[8] Janocha A., Milczarek A., Osek M., Turyk Z. 2010. Efektywność bakterii probiotycznych i prebiotyku w żywieniu kurcząt brojlerów. Acta Sci. Pol., Zootechnica 9 (1) : 21-30.

[9] Pirgozliev V., Rose1S. P., Ivanova S. 2019. Feed additives in poultry nutrition. Bulgarian Journal of Agricultural Science, Agricultural Academy, 25 (Suppl.1): 8- 11.

[10] Stajnder E. 2019. Wykorzystanie roślin wysokobiałkowych w żywieniu drobiu. Dział Technologii Produkcji Rolniczej i Doświadczalnictwa. MODR z s. w Karniowicach. 1-14.

[11] Świątkiewicz S., Koreleski J. 2007. Dodatki paszowe o działaniu immunomodulacyjnym w żywieniu drobiu. Medycyna Wet., 63 (11) : 1291-1295.

[12] Lipiński K., Tywończuk J., Siwicki A. 2009. Wpływ mannanoligosacharydów na status zdrowotny i jakość mięsa kurcząt brojlerów. ŻYWNOŚĆ. Nauka. Technologia. Jakość, 4 (65) : 26 – 33.

[13] Watzl B., Girrbach S., Roller M. 2005. Inulin, oligofructose and immunomodulation. Brit. J. Nutr., 93, Suppl. 1 : S49–S55.

[14] Patterson J.A., Burkholder K.M. 2003. Application of prebiotics and probiotics in poultry production. Poult. Sci., 82 : 627-631.

[15] Vidanarachchi J. K., Mikkelsen L. L., Constantinoiu C.C., Choct M., Iji P. A. 2013. Natural plant extracts and prebiotic compounds as alternatives to antibiotics in broiler chicken diets in a necrotic enteritis challenge model. Animal Production Science, 53 : 1247-1259.

[16] Haghighi H. R., Gong J., Gyles C. L., Hayes M. A., Sanei B., Parvizi P., Gisavi H., Chambers J. R., Sharif S. 2005. Modulation of antibody-madiated immune response by probiotics in chickens. Clin. Diagn. Lab. Immunol. 12:1387-1392.

[17] Ogawa T., Asai Y., Sakamoto H., Yasuda K. 2006. Oral immunoadjuvant activity of Lactobacillus casei subp. casei in dextran fed layer chicken. Brit. J. Nutr., 95 : 430-434.

[18] Hooge D.M., 2003. Dietary mannan oligosaccharides improve broiler and turkey performance: metaanalysis of pen trials around the world. Proc. of the Alltech's 19th Annual Symposium: Nutritional Biotechnology in the Feed and Food Industries. T.P. Lyons and K.A. Jacques, ed. Nottingham University Press, Loughborough, Leics, UK, 113-124.

[19] Lipiński K., Kaliniewicz J., Tywończuk J. 2011. Stasiewicz M. Wpływ dodatków probiotycznych i ziołowych na produkcyjność i jakość mięsa indyków. Roczniki Naukowe Polskiego Towarzystwa Zootechnicznego, 7 (2) : 29-35.

[20] Szkucik K., Pisarski R., Ziomek M., 2011. Wpływ wybranych ziół na profil kwasów tłuszczowych w tłuszczu kurcząt. Medycyna Wet. 67 (3) : 198-201.

[21] Grela E.R. 2020. Alternatywne dla soi pasze białkowe w żywieniu świń i drobiu. Życie Weterynaryjne. 95(8) : 480-486.

[22] Kwiecień M., Winiarska-Mieczan A., Kapica M. 2006. The influence of some herbs on chemical composition, lipid metabolism indices, ALAT and ASAT activity in broiler chickens liver. Polish Journal of Natural Sciences, 3 (Suppl) : 439-444.

[23] Kwiecień M., Winiarska-Mieczan A., 2009. Effect of addition of herbs on body weight and assessment of physical and chemical alterations In the tibia bones of broiler chickens. Journal of Elementology, 14 : 705- 715.

[24] Lee K.W., Everts H., Kappert H.J., Frehner M., Losa R., Beynen A.C. 2003. Effect of dietary essential oil components on growth performance, digestive enzymes and lipid metabolism in female broiler chickens. British Poultry Science, 44 : 450-457.

[25] Radkowska I., 2013. Wykorzystanie ziół i fitogenicznych dodatków paszowych w żywieniu zwierząt gospodarskich. Wiadomości Zootechniczne, LI(4) : 117-124.

[26] Plata K. 2019. Dodatki ziołowe w żywieniu zwierząt (antybiotykooporność). Pomorski Ośrodek Doradztwa Rolniczego w Lubaniu, : 1-12.

[27] Windisch W., Schedle K., Plitzner C., Kroismayr A., 2008. Use of phytogenic products as feed additives for swine and poultry. Journal of Animal Science, 86 : 140-148.

[28] Gardzielewska J., Majewska T., Pudyszak K., Jakubowska M. 2003. Wpływ dodatku preparatu DIGESTAROM i węgla drzewnego w żywieniu kurcząt brojlerów na jakość mięsa i jego przydatność do przechowywania. ŻYWNOŚĆ 4(37) Supl., 84-92.

[29] Si W., Gong J., Tsao R., Zhou T., Yu H., Poppe C., Johnson R., Du Z. 2006. Antimicrobial activity of essential oils and structurally related synthetic food additives towards selected pathogenic and beneficial gut bacteria. Journal of Applied Microbiology, 100 : 296-305.

[30] Hashemipour H., Kermanshahi H., Golian A., Veldkamp T. 2013. Effect of thymol and carvacrol feed supplementation on performance, antioxidant enzyme activities, fatty acid composition, digestive enzyme activities, and immune response in broiler chickens. Poultry Science, 92 : 2059-2069.

[31] Arczewska-Włosek A., Świątkiewicz S. 2012. The effectiveness

of the herbal extracts and chitosan under conditions of the natural exposure of chickens to coccidia. Proceedings XXIV International Poultry Symposium PB WPSA: Science for poultry practice-poultry practice for science, 12-14. 09, Kołobrzeg, 204.

[32] Majewska T., Mikulski D., Święcicka-Grabowska G., Wójcik R. 2007. Wodny wyciąg czosnku w żywieniu indyków rzeźnych. Medycyna Weterynaryjna, 63(11) : 1357-1360.

[33] Bölükbasi S.C., Erhan M.K., Kaynar Ő. 2008. The effect of feeding thyme, sage and rosemary oil on laying hen performance, cholesterol and some proteins ratio of egg yolk and *Escherichia coli* count in feces. Archiv Fur Geflügelkunde, 72(5) : 231-237.

[34] Kiczorowska B., Samolińska W., Ridha Mustafa Al-Yasiry A., Winiarska-Mieczan A., Kwiecień M. 2015. Nutritional value of poultry meat produced in conventional and organic systems. Probl Hig Epidemiol., 96(3) : 598-602.

[35] Fortomaris P., Arsenos G., Tserveni-Gousi A., Yannakopoulos A. 2007. Performance and behaviour of broiler chickens as affected by the housing system. Archiv Fur Geflügelkunde, 71(3) : 97-104.

[36] Shah D. H., Seol J. W., Park S. Y., Ryu K. S., Kwon J. T., Cho M. R., Park J. H., Kang C. H., Chae J. S. 2005. Control of fowl typhoid using tissue culture medium waste after harvest of korean wild ginseng (*Panax ginseng*). J. Appl. Poultry Sci., 14 : 455-462.

[37] Waihenya R. K., Mtambo M. M., Nkwengulila G., Minga U. M. 2002. Efficacy of crude extract of *Aloe secundiflora* against Salmonella gallinarum in experimentally infected free-range chickens in Tanzania. J. Ethnopharmacol., 79 : 317-323.

[38] Gaweł E., Grzelak M. 2013. Koncentrat białkowo-ksantofilowy z lucerny w żywieniu zwierząt. Journal of Research and Applications in Agricultural Engineering, Vol. 58(3) :137-142.

[39] Sredanović S., Lević J., Duragić O. 2006. Alfalfa concentrate – natural color and source of protein in broiler feeding. Progress of Theoretical and Experimental Physics (PTEP), 10(1-2) : 28-32.

[40] Dong X.F., Gao W.W., Tong J.M., Jia H.Q., Sa R.N., Zhang Q. 2007. Effect of Polysavone (alfalfa extract) on abdominal fat deposition and immunity in broiler chickens. Poult Sci., 86, 1955-1959.

[41] Ognik K., Czech A. 2010. Influence of protein-xanthophylls concentrate of alfalfa (*Medicago sativa*) additive on antioxidant potential of turkeys blood. Zeszyty Naukowe Polskiego Towarzystwa Zootechnicznego, 6 : 77-86.

[42] Gornowicz E., Pietrzak M., Stanisławski D., Steppa R., Lewko L., Kryza A. 2017. Charakterystyka jakości mięsa kurcząt rzeźnych odchowywanych ekologicznie i intensywnie. Roczniki Naukowe Polskiego Towarzystwa Zootechnicznego, 13(3) : 33-41.

[43] Kierończyk B., Długosz J., Rawski M., Urbański J., Józefiak D. 2016. Zastosowanie owadów w żywieniu drobiu. Polskie Drobiarstwo, 4 : 8-13.

[44] Smith R., Prior R. 2013. Insects as sustainable sources of protein. PROteINSECT. Work Package 5: Pro-Insect Platform in Europe. Minerva. Deliverable 5.1 - Mapping Exercise Report with regard to current Legislation & Regulation: Europe and Africa & China.

[45] Józefiak D., Józefiak A., Kierończyk B., Rawski M., Świątkiewicz S., Długosz J., Engberg R.M. 2016. Insects-a natural nutrient source for poultry - a review. Annals of Animal Sciene. DOI: 10.1515/aoas-2016-0010.

[46] Gilewski R., Wężyk S. 2017. Żywienie brojlerów w przyszłości. Ogólnopolski informator drobiarski. 314(11) : 8-20.

[47] Radziun B. 2019. Owady jako źródło białka w paszach dla zwierząt. PODRw Lubaniu, 1-4.

[48] Kaczmarowski M. 2019. Gatunki owadów zaliczone do zwierząt gospodarskich w Unii Europejskiej. Życie Weterynaryjne, 94(2) : 158-161.

Chapter 2

Phytogenic Feed Additives as An Alternative to Antibiotic Growth Promoters in Poultry Nutrition

Jet Saartje Mandey and Florencia Nery Sompie

Abstract

Phytoadditives in animal nutrition have attracted a lot of attention for their potential role as alternatives to antibiotic growth promoters. Phytoadditives are feed additives originated from plants or botanicals that are used in poultry nutrition. This chapter provides an overview about the potency of alternative additive from plants as a basis for exploring it as a phytoadditive for poultry. These substances are derived from herbs, spices, and other plants and their extracts. They are natural, less toxic, residue free and ideal feed additives for poultry when compared to synthetic antibiotics. There efficacy of phytogenic applications in poultry nutrition depends on several factors, such as composition and feed inclusion level of phytogenic preparations, bird genetics, and overall diet composition. Addition of 100 mg/kg feed essential oils consist of carvacrol, thymol and limonene in matrix encapsulation improved performance and apparent ideal digestibility of nutrients of broiler chickens. Besides enhancing performance, phytogenic also has antioxidant, the effects of which are associated with essential oils (EOs) and their components. Administration of eucalyptus and peppermint oil blends by oral (0.25 ml/L drinking water) and spray route (0.1 ml/20 ml water) reduced Newcastle disease infection in broilers. Phytoadditives have antimicrobial, antifungal, antiviral, antitoxigenic, antiparasitic and insecticidal properties. The benefits of using phytoadditives in poultry nutrition are increased feed intake, stimulation of digestion, increased growth performance, reduced incidence of disease, improved reproductive parameters, feed efficiency, profitability. Based on the latest scientific findings presented in this chapter, the following main conclusions have been drawn that phytomolecule and that bioactives have potential to be developed as an alternative additive for poultry, and that promote health.

Keywords: antioxidant activity, nutrition, phytoadditive, phytogenic, broiler chickens, layers

1. Introduction

All animals need to receive a nutritious diet in order to maintain good health and production. Diets for poultry generally consist of cereal grain and a protein sources. The nutritional quality of a feed depends on feed presentation, antinutritional factors, microbial contamination, palatability, digestibility, and intestinal healthfulness, and a variety of feed additives are important too.

Feed additives are nonnutritive products added to the based diet, and are minor components of the animal diet. Feed additives are products used in animal nutrition for the purposes of improving the quality of feed and the quality of food from animal origin, improve the animal's performance and health, e.g. providing enhanced digestibility of the feed materials. Feed additives promote ingestion, absorption, assimilation of nutrients, growth, and health by affecting the physiological processes, such as immune function and stress resistance. Feed additives include immunostimulants, prebiotics, probiotics, acidifiers, essential oils, or others. Some of the commonly feed additives in animal diets include enzymes, pro- and prebiotics, antioxidants, antibiotic growth promoters, and coloring agents. These ingredients are aimed to enhance digestibility or availability of nutrients, improve animal gut health and food product quality, and promote environmental protection.

Alternative feed additives (phytogenic feed additives = phytoadditives) derived from herbs, spices or aromatic plants are have gained considerable attention in the recent years (**Figure 1**). Phytogenics were classified according to botanical origin, processing, and composition. For example, phytogenic feed additives like herbs and non-woody flowering plants have medicinal properties; spices, herbs with an intensive smell or taste, commonly added to human food; essential oils, aromatic oily liquids derived from plant materials such as flowers, leaves, fruits, and roots; and oleoresins, extracts derived by non-aqueous solvents from plant material. This chapter aimed to review the phytogenic feed additives as an alternative to antibiotic growth promoters in poultry nutrition.

Phytoadditive			Major Component and Potency
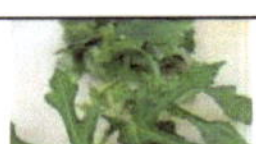	Gedi (*Abelmoschus manihot L. Medik*) leaves	Parts of plant (leaves)	flavonoid, phenolic compound, antioxidant activity
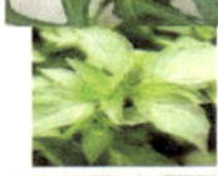	Lemon basil (*Ocimum × citriodorum*) leaves		caffeic acid, flavonoid, antioxidant and antimicrobial activity
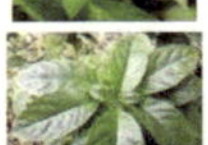	Leilem (*Clerodendrum minahassae* L.) leaves		flavonoid, phenolic compound, antioxidant activity
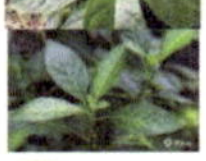	Bitter leaves (*Vernonia amygdalina*)		flavonoid, phenolic compound, antioxidant activity
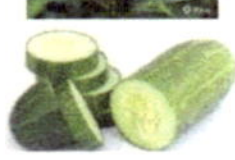	Cucumber (*Cucumis sativus*) seeds	Parts of plant (seeds)	lipid lowering, antioxidant activity
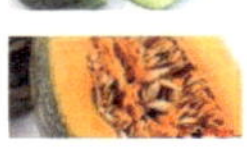	Pumpkin (*Cucurbita moschata*) seeds		phenolic compound, antioxidant activity
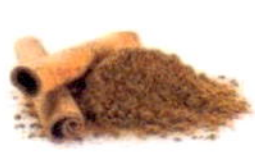	Cinnamon (*Cinnamomum verum*)	Spices	Cinnamic acid and cinnamaldehyde, antioxidant activity
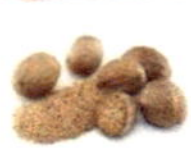	Nutmeg (*Myristica fragrans*)		Essential oils
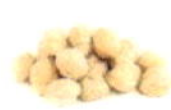	Candlenut (*Aleurites moluccanus*)		polyphenols content
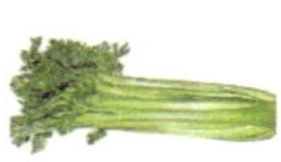	Celery (*Apium graveolens*)	Aromatic plants	natural antioxidants (especially vitamins, flavonoids, and unsaturated fatty acids)
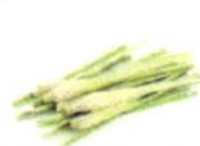	Lemongrass (*Cymbopogon citratus*)		antioxidant activity

Figure 1.
Several alternative Phytoadditive from herbs, spices, and aromatic plants.

2. Phytogenic feed additive in poultry

Phytogenics, also referred to as plant secondary metabolites, phytochemicals, phytobiotics or botanicals, are plant-derived products/extracts and include a wide range of substances such as herbs, spices, and essential oils reported to exhibit growth promoting and/or therapeutic properties [1, 2]. The use of phytogenics as an alternative prevent the risk of pathogens resistant to antibiotics in poultry. The ability of phytogenics to contribute to the health of poultry production is well documented, however, the exact mechanisms by which phytogenic exerts its effects remain speculative [3, 4].

Plant derived products are residue-free unlike synthetic antibiotics and are also considered safe to be used as the ingredients in the food industry as well as in animal diet as an ideal growth promoter. The herbs and plant extracts used as feed additives include many different bioactive ingredients such as alkaloids, bitters, flavonoids, glycosides, mucilage, saponins, tannins phenolics, polyphenols, terpenoids, polypeptide, thymol, cineole, linalool, anethole, allicin, capsaicin, allylisothiocyanate, and piperine [5]. The effects expected of herbs and plant extracts are also various. Other factors that influence the potency of the phytogenic may include the plant parts, the genetic, age and harvest time of the plant, and extraction method [6].

The concerns about antibiotic resistance cause it to explore alternatives antibiotics which have growth-promoting effects. This antibiotics as feed additive is expected not to induce resistance to bacteria and have no potential side effects to animals. Some feed additives, pro/prebiotics, organic acids, enzymes and phytogenics, are used as a replacement for AGP [7–10]. Phytogenic feed additive has been reported to enhance performance, feed conversion ratio, carcass meat safety and quality in animals [9, 11]. Besides enhancing performance, phytogenic also has antioxidant property, the effects of which are associated with essential oils (EOs) and their components [12]. Phytogenic has beneficial effects on nutrient utilization possibly by stimulating digestive enzymes and improves gastrointestinal morphology [10].

Several alternatives to AGP have been proposed, such as organic acids, probiotics, herbs and herbal products. Organic acids and medicinal plants as natural feed additives are recently used in poultry diet to enhance the performance and the immune response of birds. Yang et al. [13] reported that the lipophilic nature of phytogenic compounds limits the efficient delivery of these compounds to the gut. This problem could be resolved by microencapsulation and combination with other compounds. Hafeez et al. [14] reported that 100 mg/kg feed essential oils matrix encapsulation with active ingredients carvacrol, thymol and limonene improved performance and apparent ideal digestibility of nutrients of broiler chickens.

The use of feed additives to improve the efficiency of growth, eggs production, prevent disease and improve feed utilization is a strategy to improve the efficiency of the poultry industry.

The use and development of enzymes, phytogenics, prebiotics and probiotics has gained momentum in poultry feeding. Enzymes are of interest to improve nutrients digestibility, particularly in young animals. Phytogenics are an alternative to in-feed antibiotics to prevent the risk of developing pathogens. Probiotic which is consist of one single strain or a combination of several strains of bacteria, and prebiotics which are non-digestible food ingredients, such as fructooligosaccharides, xylooligosaccharides, mannanoligosaccharides and galactooligosaccharides, are also used in feeds to protect poultry against pathogens. Needs to be understanding how these additives can be used to improve the efficiency of poultry production [15]. In **Figure 1** showed the several alternative phytoadditive from herbs, spices, and aromatic plants.

According to Abudabos et al. [16] dietary supplementation of different feed additives in 10 treatments (**Table 1**) improved growth performance and gut health by mitigating the negative effect of the disease.

Treatment	**p Value**						
	FI(g)	**BWG (g)**	**FCR**	**PEF**	**Villus height (μm)**	**Villus width (μm)**	**Total area (mm^2)**
Negative Control							
Positive Control							
T1							
T2							
T3	0.0001	0.0001	0.0001	0.0001	NS	0.0001	NS
T4							
T5							
T6							
T7							
T8							

T1: Maxus; T2: CloSTAT; T3: Sangrovit; T4: CloSTAT +Sangrovit; T5: Gallipro Tect; T6: Saccharomyces boulardii; T7: Oregano; T8: Varium.

Table 1.
The effects of treatments on feed intake (FI), body weight gain (BWG), feed conversion ratio (FCR), body weight (BW), performance efficiency factor (PEF), villi height (L), width (W), and villi total area (TA) of broiler chickens [16].

Antimicrobial growth promoters (AGPs) are the most frequently used chemical agents, which enhance feed conversion ratio and reduce chicken mortality [17]. The use of AGPs has been associated with acquired resistance and meat residues that jeopardize human health [18]. Consequently, in many advanced countries, the unlimited use of these AGPs has been discouraged, therefore, the poultry producers are looking for alternative to antibiotics such as phytogentics [16, 19]. These natural products mostly originate from plant sources are potent source of improved growth performance and health in broilers [20–22]. Plants derived extract, polyphenol and oils enhance the absorption of nutrients, secrete the digestive enzymes, improve the immune response and antioxidant status in broiler [23].

The essential oils (EOs) present in phytogenic feed additive (PFA) contain most of the bioactive substances of the plant which include carvacrol, eugenol, thymol, capsaicin, cineole and so on are well known for their antibacterial, antifungal, antiviral and anticoccidial properties [24, 25]. In a study, supplementation of phytogenic feed additive 250 mg/kg EOs of thyme and anise improved growth performance, reduced blood total cholesterol, and also inhibited *C. perfringens* and *E. coli* prolification in small and large intestines in broiler chicks under oral *C. perfringens* 5 mL (10^7 cfu/mL) culture challenge [26]. Administration of eucalyptus and peppermint oil blends by oral (0.25 mL/L drinking water for 12 hours/day) and spray route (0.1 mL/20 mL water/10 birds) reduced Newcastle disease infection in broilers [27].

Since long time herbal and traditional plants had been used to prevent and control many diseases and health problems on a small scale such as in heavy metals toxicity [28, 29], ectoparasites [30], reproductive and renal toxicity [31, 32], heat stress [28, 29], and viral disease [33, 34]. People in the world are now aware of the advantageous use of natural derived products such as and botanicals [33, 35]; microalgae [36–43], and rare earth elements [42], over synthetic drugs and chemical in term of lower cost, toxicity and adverse effects and very low resistance [44].

Herbal medicine is gaining more importance in the anti-influenza research owing to their widespread availability and easy application in the diet [45].

Interesting in alternative products with antibacterial or anti-inflammatory activities has increased. Such products usually searching for among secondary plant metabolites, are flavonoids [46, 47]. Flavonoids are the largest and the most important single group of polyphenols. Molecular mechanisms of polyphenol health-promoting properties were related to their antioxidant properties [48]. Natural substances (flavonoids, polyphenols and isoflavones) in plants present an anti-inflammatory and antioxidative activity. Inflammatory reactions play a role of many conditions related to respiratory system [49].

The poultry industry plays a vital role in supply of healthy meat products to the public. Botanical extract were positively influenced broiler physiology, improved meat quality aid health-beneficial meat production shown by the higher meat content of essential amino acids, lower meat levels of saturated fatty acids and higher level of UFA, MUFA, PUFA, and omega-3 and optimal fatty acid ratios. These natural botanical antioxidants are good modulators of amino acid and fatty acid contents in broiler meat [50]. The supplementation of plant-derived (basil and chamomile) rich in antioxidant compounds in broiler feeds improved growth parameters in broiler chicks and had blood lipid-lowering effects by reduced serum levels of total lipids, triglycerides, and cholesterol [51]. Hashemipour et al. [52] reported dietary supplementation of phytogenic product containing an equal mixture of thymol and carvacrol at 4 levels (0, 60, 100, and 200 mg/kg of diet), thymol + carvacrol enhanced BW gain and feed efficiency, and reduced feed intake. Also, the additive increased antioxidant and digestive enzyme activities and improved immune response, which may beneficially affect health and performance of broiler chickens.

For the alleviation of diseases, modulation of immune response has been great pointed to researchers [53]. The supplementation of poultry feed with anise as reported to improve lymphocyte counts [54]. The increase in IgG in broilers was noted with the inclusion of 0.1% of herb mixture consisting *Phlomis umbrosa* Turez, *Cynancum wilfordii* Hem, *Zingiber officinale* Rosc and *Platycodi radix* in broiler [55].

Some studies reported that administration of *Withania somnifera* extract 10–30 g/L to broiler chicks improve their feed intake, body weight gain, hematological profile and immunological status [56]. That *W. somnifera* root extract has antiviral property against Infectious Bursal Disease Virus [57]. Studied on the immunomodulatory potential of the herbs such as *W. somnifera*, *T. cordifolia* and *A. indica* were suggested to combat depressed hematological parameters and stunted growth in chicks during chicken infectious anemia virus (CIAV) [58].

Alhajj et al. [59] reported that supplementation 1 or 2 g of star anise/kg of diet improve body weight, daily weight gain and feed conversion ratio. Supplementation 6 g kg^{-1} had higher antibody titers against NDV and IBV whereas the diet containing 1 g kg^{-1} had the highest antibody titers against IBDV. That Chinese star anise could be used as a natural additive to improve the immune responsiveness and performance of broiler chickens. A heat-stable encapsulated essential oils consisting of 4.5 g cinnamaldehyde and 13.5 g thymol in the diet could substitute zinc bacitracin and resulted in enhanced growth performance, production efficiency index and immune responses of broilers [60].

3. Impact of phytoadditives on the composition of digesta and its consequents on health status and performance of birds

Gut microbiota and their metabolic products improve nutrient digestion, absorption, metabolism, and overall health and growth performance of poultry [61].

Antibiotics are either synthetic drugs or are obtained from natural sources are used to kill or inhibit the growth of microorganisms in a broad sense, but these antibiotics also play some beneficial role in the gut. Administering 0.8 mg amoxicillin per bird per day in drinking water for a period of 24 h to the normal early life microbial colonization of the jejunum in 1-day old chickens is important to early life microbial colonization of the gut in relation to immune development and to modulate the early life colonization of 'beneficial' microbiota [62]. Because antibiotics reduce the gut microbiota and their toxic metabolites, antibiotics have been widely incorporated into the poultry industry for decades. Now, the use as the prophylactic dose in animal feed has been banned in some jurisdictions [61].

Feed additives that can modulate the broiler gastrointestinal tract (GIT) and provide benefit to bird performance and health have recently received more interest for commercial applications. They can also limit foodborne pathogen establishment in bird flocks by modifying the gastrointestinal microbial population. Prebiotics are known as non-digestible carbohydrates that stimulate the growth of beneficial bacteria, thus improving the overall health of the host. Other gut activities occur due to the presence of the prebiotic, including generation of short-chain fatty acids and lactic acid as microbial fermentation products, a decreased rate of pathogen colonization, and potential bird health benefits [63].

The emergence of antibiotic resistance in pathogens identified as public health risks has led to the curtailment of routine antibiotic supplementation for agricultural use and outright banning in some parts of the world [64, 65]. A wide range of feed additives have been explored for potential application in poultry including phytobiotics, organic acids, probiotics and prebiotics, and these have been extensively discussed in a number of reviews [66–70].

Prebiotics, as being indigestible by the host, are hydrolyzed and utilized by the GIT microorganisms present in various compartments of the avian GIT. Dietary fibers as undigested dietary material generally transit through the upper parts of the GIT and reach the ceca as substrates for the resident cecal microbial population [71]. Foodborne pathogens such as *Salmonella* can also reside in the ceca and the production of SCFA would presumably be antagonistic to their presence [69, 72]. The ceca have several potential roles associated with bird function, including electrolyte and water reabsorption [71].

To improved GIT and host health benefits, prebiotics offer a dietary means to select for GIT bacteria that can potentially serve as a barrier for colonization by foodborne pathogens such as *Campylobacter* and *Salmonella* [72–74]. Low energy content in the diet can decrease broiler performance, lower AME value and nutrient digestibility. Supplementing phytonutrients to a low energy diet can maintain FCR thus increase economic profit of broilers apparently via improved gut health [75].

Phytogenics and probiotics have the ability to stabilize the intestinal environment and provide positive advantages to the colonization and proliferation of Lactobacilli and reducing pathogenic organisms. Also the use of medicinal plants is safer and cheaper. It could also serve as a way of bridging the gap between food safety and production as well as reducing mortality in animals [76].

3.1 Impact of phytoadditive on digestibility of nutrients

Beneficial effects on nutrient digestibility using different phytogenic feed additive (PFA) in some previous researches have been observed in poultry [10, 77]. The reason for improvement in nutrient absorption may be partly explained due to stimulation in secretions of saliva, bile and enhanced enzyme activity [78]. The improved nutrient digestibility consequently enhances the health status of animals.

The inclusion of 100 and 200 mg/kg thymol and carvacrol in broiler chickens' diet improved villus surface, villus height, villus height to crypt depth and muscular layer of jejunum and ileum [52]. The addition of *Euphorbia hirta* (7.5 g/kg) increased the villus height compared to the control birds [79]. The dietary supplementation with 2.0 and 2.5% of *Boswellia serrata* resin to broiler led to a significant increase in the length of the duodenum and total intestine [80].

Feeding broilers a diet supplemented with 200 mg/kg EO from peppermint led to the increase of crude protein digestibility [81]. Pirgozliev et al. [4] defined that phytogenic did not affect dietary ME, but caused a significant improvement in the utilization of dietary energy, which did not always relate to growth performance. Inclusion of menthol and anethole meal at 150 mg/kg in diet had no effect to performance and apparent ileal absorption of phosphorus, however, addition of essential oils of caravacol, thymol, and limonene in encapsulated form 100 mg/kg improved performance and apparent digestibility of nutrients in broilers possibly due to improved secretion of digestive enzymes [14]. Mandey et al. [82] (**Table 2**) reported that broiler chickens which got gedi leaves juice in drinking water had the value of AME for 20 and 30 ml/L were significantly lower than control diet and 10 ml/L.

Several studies documented the use of PFA as a growth promoter [83, 84]. The supplementation of fenugreek seeds (1, 2 and 3%) significantly improved feed conversion ratio of broiler chickens [85]. Another study reported that supplementation of 1 or 2 g of anise seed in broilers diet improved body weight, daily weight gain and feed conversion ratio but had no effect on feed intake [86]. The use of herbal mixture supplement in diet had a beneficial effect in the treated chicks, improved egg productivity, vitality and health condition [87].

Dietary supplementation with thymeoil extract, especially at the level of 100 ppm, can improve immunological responses of broiler chicks [88]. The supplementation of chicken diet with extracts Curcuma and Scutelleria effectively decrease gut inflammation and increase chicken performance [89]. Using 2.5% wood vinegar in quails diet increased weight gain, decreased feed conversion ratio and increased production efficiency factor. Addition of 2.5% wood vinegar in quails diet is recommended [90]. Al-Kassie et al. [91] reported that the inclusion of mixture of hot red pepper and black pepper at a level of 0.75 and 1% in the diets significantly improved the dressing percentage of broilers.

The feed supplemented with thyme essential oil at 100 mg/kg resulted in improved dressing yield and cut up parts of carcass viz. breast yield, thigh yield and

Variables	**Treatments in Drinking Water (DW)**				***P value***
	0 mL/L DW	**10 mL/L DW**	**20 mL/L DW**	**30 mL/L DW**	
AME (Kcal/kg)	2844 ± 81.44c	2775 ± 139.60c	2534 ± 27.90b	2081 ± 108.79a	<.001
NR (g)	6.4 ± 0.51	6.1 ± 0.65	4.7 ± 0.11	2.7 ± 0.38	
AMEn (Kcal/kg)	2788 ± 77.00c	2722 ± 134.20c	2488 ± 28.37b	2057 ± 105.50a	<.001
ACP Digestibility	55.2 ± 4.29b	62.7 ± 6.61c	54.5 ± 1.22b	34.9 ± 4.70a	<.001
ACF Digestibility (%)	42.1 ± 5.55b	43.9 ± 9.93b	40.8 ± 1.58b	28.7 ± 5.14a	0.020

Source: Mandey et al. [82]; [a,b,c] the difference between means with different superscript letters in the same row is significant ($P<0.05$)

Table 2.
Effect of Gedi leaves juice in drinking water on nutrients digestibility.

back yield. However, giblet and thigh yield were not affected by addition of different doses of thyme oil in broilers diet [92]. Ragaa et al. [93] reported significantly higher breast yield and thigh yield in birds fed diet thyme 1 g/kg. The improved carcass traits might be due to utilization of nutrient from diet. Amino acids especially lysine is critical for muscle development such as breast muscle.

Broilers fed diets including EOs in150 mg/kg of the diet significantly boosted BWG compared to broilers fed the control diet [94]. The supplementation of EOs significantly increased dressing percentage [95]. Yang et al. [6] reported improvements in FCR with EO supplementation. Supplementation of Chinese herbs extract in drinking water improve growth performance, blood biochemistry parameters, immune organ weight and immune indexes of broiler [96]. Phyo et al. [97] also observed the effect of dietary garlic and thyme seed supplementation on the production performance and gut microbial population of broiler chickens. The diet with cucumber in drinking water up to 30 g per liter water (**Table 3**) was significantly decreased abdominal fat percentage, increased blood LDL-cholesterol and feed conversion value, but were no affected to final body weight, giblet, the value of blood HDL-cholesterol, and kept the good value of carcass percentage [98].

Aloe vera and clove supplementation improved the dressing percentage and breast weight without adversely affecting the meat composition and serum enzymes. These can be used as a growth promoter in Japanese quails [99]. The inclusion of medicinal herbs, spices, vegetables, plants, seeds, and edible fungi, as ingredients of natural origin, in diet of Japanese quail improved carcass and meat quality [100].

The phytobiotics compounds such as alkaloids, anthraquinones, flavonoids, tannins, steroids and saponins in guava, avocado and malunggay leaves extract is beneficial as alternative feed additives for enhancing the growth of broiler chicks in the poultry industry. Thus, could possibly eliminate the chemical residues that may cause harmful effect to the health of the consuming public [101].

Besides immune enhancing, antimicrobial, and performance enhancing effects, phytogenics also have antioxidant property. The excellent plant derived

Variables	Treatments				SEM	p Value
	0 g CSJ	10 g CSJ	20 g CSJ	30 g CSJ		
Feed Intake (g)	2144.64	2048.24	2041.36	2039.78	21.42	.23
Average Feed Intake (g)	76.59	73.15	72.49	72.85	.76	.25
Water Intake (ml)	4285	4298	4279	4290	.71	.56
Slaughter Weight (g)	1249.97	1251.20	1273.60	1300.10	14.21	.59
Weight Gain (g)	1131.89	1137.68	1159.68	1187.78	14.21	.70
Carcass Weight (g)	764.8	787.4	780.8	798.2	9.07	.65
Carcass Percentage (%)	66.78	67.60	67.33	67.74	.34	.80
FCR	1.89^{a}	1.80^{ab}	1.76^{ab}	1.72^{b}	.02	.07
Abdominal Fat (%)	2.47^{a}	2.09^{b}	2.05^{b}	1.94^{b}	.07	.02
Total Cholesterol	118.4	120.4	118.8	112.0	2.29	0.62
HDL-Cholesterol	94.4	99.8	99.0	99.0	0.89	0.13
LDL-Cholesterol	17.2**a**	20.6^{b}	29.4**c**	28.4**c**	1.28	0.00
Triglyceride	29.8	28.2	24.8	24.2	1.07	0.19

Notes: CSJ = cucumber seed juice; ^{a,b,c} the difference between means with different superscript letters in the same row is significant ($P<0.05$).

Table 3.
Effect of treatments in drinking water on the performance of broiler chickens [98].

antioxidants are obtained from rosemary, olive leaves, thyme, marjoram, sage, oregano, etc. [61]. Some other common herbs, spices and fruits that have antioxidant property are ginger, turmeric, garlic, plum, pine bark extract, berries, pomegranate, caraway, cinnamon, clove. The effects of which are associated with EOs and their components [102, 103]. The demand for natural antioxidants in food is increasing due to their health benefits against oxidative stress and several diseases [104–106].

The oxidative stability of meat obtained from broilers, hens or turkeys in a series of studies have been reported to increase with the use of dietary supplementation of EOs. Dietary supplementation of 100 mg/kg EO blends with 5% carvacrol, 3% cinnamaldehyde and 2% capsicum oleoresin as active constituents improved the concentration of antioxidants in the liver of broiler chicken [107].

The supplementation of thymol (80 mg/animal/day) helped to reduce fear responses in quail when exposed to stressful situations [108]. Study by Ghazaghi et al. [109] noted that supplementation of *Mentha spicata* (1–4%) in the diet improved meat quality of Japanese quail. The study on the effects of PFA on egg quality is limited and variable. Abdel-Wareth and Lohakare [110] reported that 20 g/kg dry peppermint leaves in diet of laying hens can be used as an effective feed additive to improve performance.

The use of antibiotics has been minimized and replaced by effective dietary supplements such as probiotics and/or prebiotics that are claimed to enhance growth and positively modulate the immune response. The economic analysis data obtained from probiotic studies in broilers indicated that probiotic supplementation may not always be more feasible and economical to obtain maximum profitability from broiler production and hence further research in the field is currently ongoing [111]. Herbs, spices, and various other plant extracts are being evaluated as alternatives to antibiotics and some do have growth promoting effects, antimicrobial properties, and other health-related benefits [112].

Phytogenic feed additives should be used as an alternative feed additives in poultry production to maximize the overall performance of poultry because of they have no side effects, residual effects, non-hazardous and eco-friendly [113].

4. Conclusion

Based on the results presented in this chapter, the following main conclusions can be drawn:

1. Phytoadditives are natural, less toxic, residue free and ideal feed additives for poultry when compared to synthetic antibiotics.

2. Phytoadditives have antimicrobial, antifungal, antiviral, antitoxigenic, antiparasitic and insecticidal properties.

3. Besides immune enhancing, antimicrobial, and performance enhancing effects, phytogenics also have antioxidant property.

4. The benefits of using phytoadditives in poultry nutrition are increased feed intake, stimulation of digestion, increased growth performance, reduced incidence of disease, improved reproductive parameters and feed efficiency.

5. That phytomolecule and that bioactives have potential to be developed as an alternative additive for poultry, and that promote health.

Author details

Jet Saartje Mandey* and Florencia Nery Sompie
Animal Nutrition Department, Animal Husbandry Faculty, University of Sam Ratulangi, Manado, North Sulawesi, Indonesia

*Address all correspondence to: jetsm_fapet@yahoo.co.id

References

[1] Bravo D, Pirgozliev V, Rose SP. A mixture of carvacrol, cinnamaldehyde, and capsicum oleoresin improves energy utilization and growth performance of broiler chickens fed maize-based diet. Journal of Animal Science 2014;**92**: 1531-1536

[2] Pirgozliev V, Beccaccia A, Rose SP. Partitioning of dietary energy of chickens fed maize- or wheat-based diets with and without a commercial blend of phytogenic feed additives. Journal Animal Science. 2015a;**93**:1695e702

[3] Karadas F, Pirgozliev V, Rose SP, Dimitrov D, Oduguwa O, Bravo D. Dietary essential oils improve the hepatic antioxidative status of broiler chickens. British Poultry Science. 2014; **55**(3):329-334

[4] Pirgozliev V, Bravo D, Mirza MW, Rose SP. Growth performance and endogenous losses of broilers fed wheat based diets with and without essential oils and xylanase supplementation. Poultry Science. 2015b;**94**:1227-1232

[5] Al-Yasiry ARM, Kiczorowska Frankincense–therapeutic properties. Postep. Hig.Med. Dosw. 2016;**70**: 380-391

[6] Yang X, Long F, Xin H, Yang C, Yang X. Impact of essential oils and organic acids on the growth performance, digestive functions and immunity of broiler chickens. Animal Nutrition Journal. 2018;**4**:388-393

[7] Bedford MR, Cowieson AJ. Exogenous enzymes and their effects on intestinal microbiology. Animal Feed Science Technology. 2012;**173**: 76-85

[8] Gong J, Yin F, Hou Y, Yin Y. Chinese herbs as alternatives to antibiotics in feed for swine and poultry production: Potential and challenges in application. Canadian Journal Animal Science. 2014;**94**:223-241

[9] Dhama K, Latheef SK, Mani S, Samad HA, Kartik K, Tiwari R, Khan RU, Alagawany M, Farag MR, Alam GM, Laudadio V, Tufarelli V. Multiple beneficial applications and modes of action of herbs in poultry health and production – A review. International Journal Pharmacology. 2015;**11**:152-176

[10] Upadhaya SD, Kim SJ, Kim IH. Effects of gel-based phytogenic feed supplement on growth performance, nutrient digestibility, blood characteristics and intestinal morphology in weanling pigs. Journal Applied Animal Research. 2016;**44**:384-389

[11] Dhama K, Chakraborty S, Tiwari R, Verma AK, Saminathan M, Amarpal Malik YS, Nikousefat Z, Javdani M, Khan RU. 2014. A concept paper on novel technologies boosting production and safeguarding health of humans and animals. Research Opinion Animal Veterinary Science. 2014;**4**:353-370

[12] Alagawany M, Ali Ashour E, Reda FM. Effect of dietary supplementation of garlic (*Allium sativum*) and turmeric (*Curcuma longa*) on growth performance, carcass traits, blood profile and oxidative status in growing rabbit. Annual Animal Science. 2016;**16**:489-505

[13] Yang C, Chowdhury MAK, Hou Y, Gong J. Phytogenic compounds as alternatives to in-feed antibiotics: potentials and challenges in application. Pathogens. 2015;**4**:137-156

[14] Hafeez A, Ma¨nner K, Schieder C†, Zentek J. Effect of supplementation of phytogenic feed additives (powdered vs. encapsulated) on performance and nutrient digestibility in broiler chickens. Poultry Science. 2016;**95**:622-629

[15] Pirgozliev V, Rose SP, Ivanova S.2019. Feed additives in poultry nutrition. Bulgarian Journal of Agricultural Science. 2019;**25**(Suppl. 1):8-11

[16] Abudabos AM, Hussein EOS, Ali MH, Al-Ghadi MQ†. The effect of some natural alternative to antibiotics on growth and changes in intestinal histology in broiler exposed to Salmonella challenge. Poultry Science. 2019;**98**: 1441-1446

[17] Khan RU, Naz S, Nikousefat Z, Tufarelli V, Laudadio V. Thymus vulgaris: alternative to antibiotics in poultry feed. Worlds Poultry Science Journal. 2012;**68**:401-408

[18] Ayisi CL, Zhao J, Rupia EJ. Growth performance, feed utilization, body and fatty acid composition of Nile tilapia (*Oreochromis niloticus*) fed diets containing elevated levels of palm oil. Aquaculture Fish. 2017;**2**:67-77

[19] Alzawqari MH, Al-Baddany AA, Al-Baadani HH, Al-hidary IA, Khan RU, Aqil GM, Abdurab A. Effect of feeding dried sweet orange (*Citrus sinensis*) peel and lemon grass (*Cymbopogon citratus*) leaves on growth performance, carcass traits, serum metabolites and antioxidant status in broiler during the finisher phase. Environmental Science Pollution Research. 2016;**23**:1707717082

[20] Chand N, Faheem H, Khan RU, Qureshi MS, Al-hidary IA, Abudabos AM. Anticoccidial effect of mananoligosacharide against experimentally induced coccidiosis in broiler. Environmental Science Pollution Research. 2016;**23**:14414-14421

[21] Rahman S, Khan S, Chand N, Sadique U, Khan RU. 2017. In vivo effects of Allium cepa L. on the selected gut microflora and intestinal histo-morphology in broiler. Acta Histo-chemistry. 2017;**119**:446-450

[22] Abudabos AM, Alyemni AH, Dafallah YM, Khan RU. The effect of phytogenic feed additives to substitute in-feed antibiotics on growth traits and blood biochemical parameters in broiler chicks challenged with *Salmonella typhimurium*. Environmental Science Pollution Research. 2016;**23**:24151-24157

[23] Tehseen M, Tahir M, Khan RU, Jabbar A, Ahmad B, Ahsan T, Khan MS, Khan S, Abudabos AM. Additive effect of Nigella sativa and Zingiber officinale herbal mixture on performance and cholesterol profile in broiler. Phillipine Agriculture Science. 2016;**99**:408-413

[24] Farag MR, Alagawany M, Tufarelli V. In vitro antioxidant activities of resveratrol, cinnamaldehyde and their synergistic effect against cyadox-induced cytotoxicity in rabbit erythro-cytes. Drug Chemistry Toxicology. 2016;**17**:1-10

[25] Patil KR, Patil CR. Anti-inflammatory activity of bartogenic acid containing fraction of *Barringtonia racemosa* Roxb in acute and chronic animal models of inflammation. Journal Traditional Complementary Medicine. 2016;**7**(1): 86-93

[26] Cho JH, Kim HJ, Kim IH. Effects of phytogenic feed additive on growth performance, digestibility, blood metabolites, intestinal microbiota, meat color and relative organ weight after oral challenge with *Clostridium perfringens* in broilers. Livestock Science. 2014;**160**: 82-88

[27] Awaad MHH, Afify MAA, Zoulfekar SA, Mohammed FF, Elmenawy MA, Hafez HM. Modulating effect of peppermint and eucalyptus essential oils on vVND infected chickens. Pakistan Veterinary Journal. 2016;**36**: 350-355

[28] Khafaga AF, El-Hack MEA, Taha AE, Elnesr SS, Alagawany M. The potential modulatory role of herbal additives against Cd toxicity in human, animal, and poultry: a review. Environmental Science Polluttion Research. 2019a;**26**:4588-4604

[29] Khafaga AF, Noreldin AE, Taha AE. The adaptogenic anti-ageing potential

of resveratrol against heat stress-mediated liver injury in aged rats: Role of HSP70 and NF-kB signalling. Journal Therm. Biology. 2019b;**83**:8-21

[30] Abbas A, Abbas RZ, Masood S, Iqbal Z, Khan MK, Saleemi MK, Raza MA, Mahmood MS, Khan JA, Sindhu ZD. Acaricidal and insecticidal effects of essential oils against ectoparasites of veterinary importance. BLACPMA. 2018;**17**: 441-452

[31] Khafaga AF, Bayad AE. Impact of *Ginkgo biloba* extract on reproductive toxicity induced by single or repeated injection of cisplatin in adult male rats. International Journal Pharmacology. 2016a;**12**: 340-350

[32] Khafaga AF, Bayad AE. Ginkgo biloba extract attenuates hematological disorders, oxidative stress and nephrotoxicity induced by single or repeated injection cycles of cisplatin in rats: Physiological and Pathological Studies. Asian Journal Animal Science. 2016b;**10**: 235-246

[33] Mahmood MS, Amir HW, Abbas RZ, Rafique A, Aslam B. Evaluation of antiviral activity of Azadirachta indica (neem) bark extract against Newcastle disease virus. Pakistan Veterinary Journal. 2018;**38**:25-28

[34] Sun N, Sun P, Xie N, Khan A. Sun Y, Fan K, Yin W, Li H. Antiviral and immunomodulatory effects of dipotassium glycyrrhizinate in chicks artificially infected with infectious bursal disease virus. Pakistan Veterinary Journal. 2018;**39**: 43-48

[35] Shah MU, Aslam A, Mustafa G, Zahid B, Imran MS. (2018). Effect of mentofin and asimirus on humoral immune response and tissue changes in infectious bursal disease vaccinated broiler birds. Pakistan Veterinary Journal. 2018;**38**:56-60

[36] Abd El-Hack ME, Alagawany M. Performance, egg quality, blood profile, immune function, and antioxidant enzyme activities in laying hens fed diets with thyme powder. Journal Animal Feed Science.2015a;**24**:127-133

[37] Abd. El-Hack ME, Mahgoub SA, Alagawany M, Dhama K. Influences of dietary supplementation of antimicrobial cold pressed oils mixture on growth performance and intestinal microflora of growing Japanese quails. International Journal Pharmacology. 2015b;**11**:689-696

[38] Abd. El-Hack M., Alagawany M., Farag M., T iwari R., Karthik K., Dhama K., Zorriehzahra J., Adel M. (2016). Beneficial impacts of thymol essential oil on health and production of animals, fish and poultry: A review. Journal Essential Oil Research. 2016a;**28**: 365-382

[39] Abd. El-Hack ME, Alagawany M, Farag MR, Tiwari R, Karthik K, Dhama K, Zorriehzahra J, Adel M. Beneficial impacts of thymol essential oil on health and production of animals, fish and poultry: A review. Journal Essential Oil Research. 2016b;**28**:365-382

[40] Abd El-Hack ME, Mahgoub SA, Hussein MM, Saadeldin IM. (2018). Improving growth performance and health status of meat-type quail by supplementing the diet with blackcumin cold-pressed oil as a natural alternative for antibiotics. Environmental Science Poultry Research. 2018;**25**:1157-1167

[41] Abd. El-Hack ME, Abdelnour SA, Taha AE, Khafaga AF, Arif M, Ayasan T, Abdel-Daim MM. Herbs as thermo-regulatory agents in poultry: An overview. Science Total Environmental. 2019;134399

[42] Abdelnour SA, Abd. El-Hack ME, Arif M, Khafaga AF, Taha AE. The application of Chlorella microalgae as a feed supplement in broiler feed. World's Poultry Science. 2019;**75**:305-318

[43] Subhani Z, Shahid M, Hussain F, Khan JA. (2018). Efficacy of *Chlorella*

pyrenoidosa to ameliorate the hepatotoxic effects of aflatoxin B1 in broiler chickens. Pakistan Veterinary Journal. 2018;**38**:13-18

[44] Karimi A, Majlesi M, Rafieian-Kopae M. Herbal versus synthetic drugs; beliefs and facts. Journal Nephropharmacology. 2015;**4**:27-30

[45] Abd. El-Hamid HS, Ellakany HF, Elbestawy AR, Seliem AA, Khalil HS. In vitro antiviral activity of commercial products of herbal extracts against highly pathogenic avian influenza (H5N1) virus. Alexandria Journal Veterinary Science. 2018;**56**:145-152

[46] Kamboh AA, Zhu WY. 2014. Individual and combined effects of genistein and hesperidin on immunity and intestinal morphometry in lipo-polysacharide-challenged broiler chickens. Poultry Science. 2014;**93**: 2175-2183

[47] Siler B, Zivkovic S, Banjanac T, Cvetkovic J, Nestorovic ZJ, Ciric A, Sokovic M, Misic D. Centauries as underestimated food additives: Antioxidant and antimicrobial potential. Food Chemistry. 2014;**147**:367-376

[48] Surai PF. Polyphenol compounds in the chicken/animal diet: From the past to the future. Journal Animal Physiology Animal Nutrition (Berlin). 2014; **98**:19-31

[49] Korbecki J, Baranowska-Bosiacka I, Gutowska I, Chlubek D. The effect of reactive oxygen species on the synthesis of prostanoids from arachidonic acid. Journal Physiology Pharmacology. 2013;**64**:409-421

[50] Waheed S, Hasnain A, Ahmad A, Tarar OM, Yaqeen Z, Ali TM. Effect of Botanical Extracts on Amino Acid and Fatty Acid Profile of Broiler Meat. Brazilian Journal of Poultry Science. 2018;**20**(3):507-516

[51] Ahmed A, Kadry M, Sadek, Ayman E. 2015. Impact of two herbal seeds supplementation on growth performance and some biochemical blood and tissue parameters of broiler chickens. Life Sciences Research. 2015;**3**:112-127

[52] Hashemipour H, Kermanshahi H, Golian A, Veldkamp T†. 2013. Effect of thymol and carvacrol feed supple-mentation on performance, antioxidant enzyme activities, fatty acid composition, digestive enzyme activities, and immune response in broiler chickens. Poultry Science. 2013;**92**:2059-2069

[53] Mahima RA, Deb R, Latheef SK, Abd. Samad H, Tiwari R, Verma AK, Kumar A, Dhama K. Immunomodulatory and therapeutic potentials of herbal, traditional/indigenous and ethno-veterinary medicines. Pakistan Journal Biology Science. 2012;**15**:754-774

[54] Soltan MA, Shewita RS, El-Katcha MI. Effects of dietary anise seeds supplementation on growth performance, immune response, carcass traits and some blood parameters of broiler chickens. International Journal Poultry Science. 2008;7:1078-1088

[55] Begum M, Hosain MM, Kim IH. Effects of the plant extract YGF251 on growth performance, meat quality, relative organ weight, nutrient digestibility and blood profiles in broiler chickens: possible role of insulin-like growth factor 1. Veterinary Medicina. 2014;**59**:415-423

[56] Mushtaq M, Durrani FR, Imtiaz N, Sadique U, Hafeez A, Akhtar S, Ahmad S. Effect of administration of Withania somnifera on some hematological and immunological profile of broiler chicks. Pakistan Veterinary Journal. 2012;**32**:70-72

[57] Pant M, Ambwani T., Umapathi V. Antiviral activity of Ashwagandha extract on infectious bursal disease virus replication. Indian Journal Science Technology. 2012;**5**:2750-2751

[58] Latheef SK, Dhama K, Wani MY, Samad HA, Barathidasan R, Tiwari R, Singh SD, Rai RB. Ameliorative effects of four herbs (*Withania somnifera*, *Tinospora cordifolia*, *Azadirachta indica* and EcareSE herbal) on the pathogenesis of chicken infectious anaemia virus. International Journal Current Research. 2013;**5**(8):2327-2331

[59] Alhajj MS, Alhobaishi M, Nabi R, Al-Mufarrej S. Immune responsiveness and performance of broiler chickens fed a diet supplemented with high levels of Chinese star anise fruit (*Illicium verum* Hook. F). Journal Animal Veterinary Advances. 2015;**14**:36-42

[60] Attia Y, Al-Harthi M, El-Kelawy M. Utilisation of essential oils as a natural growth promoter for broiler chickens. Italian Journal of Animal Science. 2019;**18**(1):10051012

[61] Yadav S, Jha R. Strategies to modulate the intestinal microbiota and their effects on nutrient utilization, performance, and health of poultry. Journal of Animal Science and Biotechnology. 2019;**10**(2):2-11

[62] Schokker D, Jansman AJ, Veninga G, De Bruin N, Vastenhouw SA, de Bree FM. Perturbation of microbiota in one-day old broiler chickens with antibiotic for 24 hours negatively affects intestinal immune development. BMC Genomics.2017;**18**(1):241

[63] Ricke SC,† Sang In Lee,† Sun Ae Kim, Si Hong Park, Zhaohao Shi. 2020. Prebiotics and the poultry gastro-intestinal tract microbiome. Poultry Science. 2020;**99**:670-677

[64] Ventola CL. The antibiotic crisis. Part 1: Causes and threats. Pharmacy & Therapeutics. 2015;**40**:227-283

[65] Van Boekel TP, Glennon EE, Chen D, Gilbert M, Robinson TP, Grenfell BT, Levin SA, Bonhoeffer S, Laxminarayan R. Reducing antimicrobial use in food animals. Science. 2017;**357**:1350-1352

[66] O'Bryan CA, Pendleton SJ, Crandall PG, Ricke SC. Potential of plant essential oils and their components in animal agriculture – in vitro studies on antibacterial mode of action. Frontier Veterinary Science. 2015;**2**:35

[67] Rivera JC, Crandall PG, O'Bryan CA, Ricke SC. Essential oils as antimicrobials in food systems – a review. Food Controlling. 2015;**54**:111-119

[68] Clavijo V, Flórez MJV. The gastrointestinal microbiome and its association with the control of pathogens in broiler chicken production: a review. Poultry Science. 2018;**97**:1006-1021

[69] Dittoe DK, Ricke SC, and Kiess AS. Organic acids and potential for modifying the avian gastrointestinal tract and reducing pathogens and disease. Frontier Veterinary Science. 2018;**5**:216

[70] Ricke SC. Impact of prebiotics on poultry production and food safety. Yale Journal Biology Medicine. 2018;**91**: 151-159

[71] Svihus B, Choct M, Classen HL. Function and nutritional roles of the avian caeca: a review. World's Poultry Science Journal. 2013;**69**:249-263

[72] Micciche AC, Foley SL, Pavlidis HO, McIntyre DR, Ricke SC. 2018. A review of prebiotics against Salmonel la in poultry: current and future potential for microbiome research application. Frontier Veterinary Science. 2018;**5**:191

[73] Ricke SC. Potential of fructooligo-saccharide prebiotics in alternative and nonconventional poultry production systems. Poultry Science. 2015;**94**: 1411-1418

[74] Kim SA, Jang MJ, Kim SY, Yang Y, Pavlidis HO, Ricke SC. Potential for prebiotics as feed additives to limit

foodborne Campylobacter establishment in the poultry gastrointestinal tract. Frontier Microbiology. 2019;**10**:91

[75] Lei Yan, Sha An, Zunzhou Lv, Zhengguo Wang, Yueming Wu, Yutao Zhu, Min Zhao, Chunhua Sun, Mingbin Lv, Zhengpeng Zhu, Yuming Gu. Effects of phytonutrients on growth performance, antioxidative status, and energy utilization of broilers fed low energy diets. Animal Nutrition. 2019;**5**: 270-277

[76] Omolere ABM and Alagbe JO. Probiotics and Medicinal Plants in Poultry Nutrition: A Review. International Journal of Family Medicine and Primary Care. 2020;**1**(4), No1020:1-5

[77] Gheisar MM, Im YW, Lee HH, Choi YI, Kim IH. Inclusion of phytogenic blends in different nutrient density diets of meat-type ducks. Poultry Science.2015;**94**(12):2952-2958

[78] Jang IS, Ko JH, Kang SY, Lee CY. Effect of commercial essential oils on growth performance, digestive enzyme activity and intestinal microflora population in broiler chickens. Animal Feed Science Technology. 2007;**134**: 304-315

[79] Hashemi SR, Zulkifli I, Davoodi H, HairBejo M, Loh TC. Intestinal histomorphology changes and serum biochemistry responses of broiler chickens fed herbal plant (Euphorbia hirta) and mix of acidifier. Iranian Journal Applied Animal Science. 2014;**4**: 95-103

[80] Kiczorowska B, Samolińska W, Al-Yasiry ARM, Kowalczyk-Pecka D. Effect of supplementation of mixtures for broiler chickens with *Boswellia serrata* on the condition of the gastrointestinal tract and rearing efficiency. Annual Animal Science. 2016;**16**:1-15

[81] Khodambashi N, Samie A, Rahmani H, Ruiz-Feria CA. The effect of peppermint essential oil and fructo-oligosaccharides, as alternatives to virginiamycin, on growth performance, digestibility, gut morphology and immune response of male broilers. Animal Feed Science Technology. 2012;**175**:57-64

[82] Mandey JS, Soetanto H, Sjofjan O, Tulung B. Digestibility and nutritional value of gedi (*Abelmoschus manihot* (l.) Medik) leaves meal in the diet of broilers. Proceeding The 6th Int. Seminar on Tropic. Anim. Prod. Yogyakarta, 20-22 October 2015. Pp. 100-104.

[83] Bartos P, Dolan A, Smutny L, Sístkova M, Celja I, Soch M, Havelka Z. Effects of phytogenic feed additives on growth performance and on ammonia and greenhouse gases emissions in growing-finishing pigs. Animal Feed Science Technology. 2016;**212**:143-148

[84] Li HN, Zhao PY, Yan L, Hossain MM, Kang J., Kim IH. Dietary phytoncide supplementation improved growth performance and meat quality of finishing pigs. Asian Australasian Journal Animal Science. 2016;**9**:1314-1321

[85] Mamoun T, Mukhtar A, Tabidi MH. Effect of fenugreek seed powder on the performance, carcass characteristics and some blood serum attributes. Advanced Research Agriculture Veteriner Science. 2014;**1**:6-11

[86] Alhajj MS, Alhobaishi M, Nabi AR, Al-Mufarrej SI. Immune responsiveness and performance of broiler chickens fed a diet supplemented with high levels of Chinese star anise fruit (*Illicium verum* Hook. F). Journal Animal Veterinary Advances. 2015;**14**:36-42

[87] Gerzilov V, Nikolov A. Petrov P, Bozakova N, Penchev G, Bochukov A. Effect of a dietary herbal mixture supplement on the growth performance, egg production and health status in chickens. J. Central European Agriculture. 2015;**16**:10-27

[88] Alipour F, Hassanabadi A, Golian A, Moghaddam HN. Effect of plant extracts derived from thyme on male broiler performance. Poultry Science 2015;**94**:2630-2634

[89] Varmuzova K, Matulova ME, Gerzova L, Cejkova D, Gardan-Salmon D,† Panh´eleux M,† Robert F,† Sisak F, Havlickova H, Rychlik I. Curcuma and Scutellaria plant extracts protect chickens against inflammation and Salmonella Enteritidis infection. Poultry Science. 2015;**94**:2049-2058

[90] Diógenes GV, Teixeira ENM, Pimenta AS, Souza JG, Moreira JA, Marinho AL, Veras A, Chemane IA. Wood vinegar from eucalyptus as an additive in broiler quail feed. International Journal Plant Animal Environmental Science. 2019;**9**(3): 164-181

[91] Al-Kassie GAM, Al-Nasrawi MAM, Ajeena SJ. Use of black pepper (*Piper nigrum*) as feed additive in broilers diet. Research Opinions in Animal and Veterinary Sciences. 2015;**1**(3):169-173

[92] Wade MR, Manwar S, Kuralkar SV, Waghmare S, Ingle VC, Hajare S. Effect of dietary thyme essential oil on carcass parameter of broiler chickens. Chemistry Science Review Letter. 2018;7(26): 669-672

[93] Ragaa NM, Korany RMS, Mohamed FF. Effect of thyme and/or organic acid dietary supplementation of broiler performance and immunity. Agriculture and Agricultural Science Procedia. 2016;**10**: 270-279

[94] Amal OA, Mukhtar AM, Mohamed KA, Ahlam AH. Use of Halfa bar essential oil (HBO (as a natural growth promoter in broiler nutrition. International Journal Poultry Science. 2013;**12**:15-18

[95] Mahmoodi BM, Ghazanfari SS, Sharifi SD. Growth performance, carcass characteristics, antibody titers and blood parameters in broiler chickens fed dietary myrtle (*Myrtus communis*) essential oil as an alternative to antibiotic growth promoter. Poultry Science Journal. 2014;**2**:37-49

[96] Rehman A, Xu Jingyi, Liu Shuang, Liu Fan, Chen Xiu Hong, He Shenghu, Zhao Hong Ji. Comparative Efficacy of Different Chinese Herbal Extracts in Broiler Production. Comparative Efficacy of Different Chinese Herbal Extracts in Broiler Production. Poultry, Fisheries & Wildlife Sciences. 2019;**7**(1), No 205

[97] Phyo HHK, Kyaw SW, Khin KL, Yezin KM, Aye AM, Khin HS. Effect of dietary garlic and thyme seed supplementation on the production performance, carcass yield and gut microbial population of broiler chickens. Journal Science Agriculture. 2017;**1**:269-274

[98] Mandey JS, Wolayan FR, Pontoh CJ, Kowel YHS. Effect of orally administrated of cucumber (*Cucumis sativus* L.) seed juice on the performance and carcass parameters of broiler chickens. IOP Conf. Series: Earth and Environmental Science. **492** (2020) 012025

[99] Tariq H, Raman Rao PV, Raghuvanshi RS, Mondal BC, Singh SK. Effect of Aloe vera and clove powder supplementation on carcass characteristics, composition and serum enzymes of Japanese quails. Veterinary World. 2015;**8**(19):664-668

[100] Sánchez RDV, Arias FJI, Martínez BdMT, Escalante AS, Urrutia GRT. 2019. Use of natural ingredients in Japanese quail diet and their effect on carcass and meat quality-A review. Asian-Australasian Journal Animal Science. 2019;**32**(11):1641-1656

[101] Mapatac LC. Potency of medicinal leaves in the growth performance of

broiler chicks. Recoletos Multidisciplinary Research Journal. 2015;**3**(1):197-206

[102] Botsoglou N, Papageorgiou G, Nikolakakis I. Effect of dietary dried tomato pulp on oxidative stability of Japanese quail meat. Journal Agriculture Food Chemisry. 2004;**52**:29822988

[103] Khan RU, Nikousefat Z, Tufarelli V, Naz S, Javdani M, Laudadio V. (2012). Garlic (*Allium sativum*) supplementation in poultry diets: Effect on production and physiology. World Poultry Science Journal. 2012;**68**:417424.

[104] Perez-Barron G, Avila-Acevedo JG, Garcia-Bores AM, Montes S, Garcia-Jimenez S, Leon-Rivera I, Rubio-Osornio M, Monroy-NoyolaA. Neuroprotective effect of *Buddleja cordata* methanolic extract inthe1-methyl-4-phenylpyridinium Parkinson's disease rat model. Journal Natural Medicine. 2015;**69**: 86-93

[105] Juadjur A, Mohn C, Schantz M, Baum M, Winterhalter P, Richling E. Fractionation of an anthocyanin-rich bilberry extract and in vitro antioxidative activity testing. Food Chemistry. 2015;**167**:418-424.

[106] Kim YS, Hwang JW, Sung SH, Jeon YJ, Jeong JH, Jeon BT, Moon SH, Park PJ. Antioxidant activity and protective effect of extract of *Celosia cristata* L. flower on tert-butyl hydroperoxide-induced oxidative hepatotoxicity. Food Chemistry. 2015;**68**:572-579.

[107] Karadas F, Pirgozliev V, Rose SP, Dimitrov D, Oduguwa O, Bravo D. Dietary essential oils improve the hepatic antioxidative status of broiler chickens. British Poultry Science. 2014;**55**:329-334.

[108] Labaque MC, Kembro JM, Luna A, Marin RH. Effects of thymol feed supplementation on female Japanese quail (*Coturnix coturnix*) behavioral fear response. Animal Feed Science Technology. 2013;**183**:67-72.

[109] Ghazaghi M, Mehri M, Kasmani FB. Effects of dietary *Mentha spicata* on performance, blood metabolites, meat quality and microbial ecosystem of small intestine in growing Japanese quail. Animal Feed Science Technology. 2014;**194**: 89-98.

[110] Abdel-Wareth AAA, Lohakare JD. (2014). Effect of dietary supplementation of peppermint on performance, egg quality, and serum metabolic profile of Hy-Line Brown hens during the late laying period. Animal Feed Science Technology. 2014;197:114-120

[111] Al-Khalaifah HS. Benefits of probiotics and/or prebiotics for antibiotic-reduced poultry. Poultry Science. 2018;**97**:3807-3815

[112] Diaz-Sanchez S, D'Souza D, Biswas D,† Irene Hanning I. 2015. Botanical alternatives to antibiotics for use in organic poultry production. Poultry Science. 2015;**94**:1419-1430

[113] Yitbarek MB. Phytogenics As Feed Additives In Poultry Production: A Review. International Journal Extensive Research. 2015;**3**:49-60

Chapter 3

Phytobiotics, a Natural Growth Promoter for Poultry

Magdalena Krauze

Abstract

Genetic advance aimed at accelerating the growth rate of slaughter birds have reduced the natural resistance of poultry to infections. It also increased susceptibility to stress, which resulted in deterioration of the welfare and productivity of poultry. Additionally, intensive poultry production poses a risk of exposure of chickens to unfavorable zoo-hygienic conditions and contamination with pathogens from the external environment (bedding, water, feed, hen house staff, sick birds in the flock). Due to the potential production losses, measures are taken to improve the health and effectiveness of bird rearing, for example by using growth stimulants and improving the composition of the gastrointestinal microbiome and improving metabolism and the work of the immune system. The addition of phytobiotics to feed or drinking water supports digestion and metabolism in the body, stimulates the growth and development of a useful microbiome, limits the multiplication and adhesion of pathogens, and improves the structure and functioning of enterocytes. The aim of this study is to present the health benefits resulting from the use of phytobiotics in poultry production, as well as to make people aware of the dangers of incompetent incorporation of herbs into feed mixtures or into drinking water. Due to the fact that not all species of animals react equally to a given plant, the selection of plant materials should be carefully considered and matched to the expected benefits. By using phytobiotics you can improve growth and performance of broiler chickens, through greatly improve digestion and nutrient assimilation. Plant additives can improve health through stimulate immunity and increase resistance to stress. Using of phitobiotics improve the quality of meat and eggs, increase the weight of valuable parts of carcass (pectoral and leg muscles) and stimulate laying. Unfortunately, due to the potentially toxic effect of an excess of certain herbs on the work of the liver, and the adverse changes in the palatability of eggs, use caution in the use some herbs e.g. of garlic, turmeric, rapeseed, alfa alfa, shiny privet or moringa.

Keywords: phytobiotic, plant additive, poultry nutrition, performance and metabolism, toxic plants

1. Introduction

The using of plant additives, the so-called phytobiotics, been known to man since ancient times, when herbs were used both in the prevention and treatment of people and farm animals. Already great civilizations: Egyptian, Chinese, Greek and Roman successfully used the specific properties of herbs and plant additives [1]. Numerous observations of the animals' reactions allowed for the use of specific herbs in the treatment of a given disease, as well as eliminating the use of those species of plants that are potentially harmful or toxic. At present, the intensive development of analytical techniques allows the identification of a whole range of biologically active substances in plants, responsible for their beneficial effects. In poultry practice can use plant additives, in both fresh and dried, fermented or freeze-dried, as well as water or alcohol extracts made on their basis [2]. In poultry rearing, in addition to basic nutrients, minerals and vitamins, feed additives are successfully used. According to the regulation of the European Parliament and of the Council [Regulation (EC) No 1831/2003], a feed additive is defined as "a substance, micro-organism or chemical substance intentionally added to a feed for the purpose of improving feed properties, meeting nutritional requirements of animals, positively influencing genetics and production animal characteristics and welfare and to increase livestock production". One such additive is phytobiotics [Regulation (EC) No 1831/2003]. The phytobiotics can expected to regulate digestive processes, support the secretion of digestive enzymes and bile, increase appetite, improve the absorption of nutrients and act to support, and also detoxification of the body. Plant supplements may, however, also act more specifically, i.e. inhibit the growth of pathogenic microorganisms, regulate the gastrointestinal microbiome, stimulate the immune, reproductive and endocrine systems, have antioxidant and antiallergic properties, accelerate wound healing, stimulate blood circulation, inhibit inflammation and promote epithelial regeneration intestines and intestinal villi, and even improve the quality of eggs or meat. The most of the active antioxidants plant, are secondary metabolites bilonging to the classes of isoprene, flavonoids and glucosinolates derivatives, and their properties could also use to shape the characteristics of food of animal origin. In practice many plant substances have been used successfully to improve egg laying, egg quality and meat quality [3–6]. The use of antibiotics as growth promoters (AGP) in livestock has been banned in year 2005, due to concerns about their residues in animal tissues and subsequent induction of bacterial resistance. Accordingly, phytobiotics are gaining in importance as possible alternatives to antibiotic growth promoters because they are natural, readily available, non-toxic and residue-free [7–9]. The phytobiotics raw materials can be herbal extracts or parts of plants (leaves, rhizomes, roots, flowers or bark, bulbs, stems, as well as fruits and seeds), in which the accumulation of biologically active substances is greatest. In addition, isolated pure bioactive substances are used, e.g. essential oils, dyes (mainly carotenoids, anthocyanins), alkaloids, glycosides, phenolic acids, phytosterols, flavonoids, etc. It is worth remembering, however, that often the desired effect of phytobiotics is not constant and fully predictable in advance [6]. Contradictory results from the use of plant additives may result from the natural variability of the composition of plant secondary metabolites, their diversity and environmental conditions for plant growth, harvest time, maturity, as well as the method and duration of conservation, storage or processing. In addition, the conditions of the analytical method required to obtain the bioactive substances themselves from plants, the method of extracting these substances from the plant are important; and possible synergism or antagonism in the case of mixtures of substances, or the presence of toxic and anti-nutritional components for a given animal species, and also microbiological contamination of plants product [1, 6]. Many researchers question results about anti-diarrheal, antiseptic, antimicrobial, and anti-inflammatory properties of plants, especially because of the variations found in biological indicators in vivo studies. It is important to note that the positive effects will depend on the animal species, the productive category, environmental conditions, and characteristics of the plant material used [2].

The aim of this study is to present the health benefits resulting from the use of phytobiotics in poultry production, as well as to make people aware of the dangers of incompetent incorporation of herbs into feed mixtures or into drinking water. Due to the fact that not all species of animals react equally to a given plant, the selection of plant materials should be carefully considered and matched to the expected benefits.

2. The influence of phytobiotics on the processes taking place in the birds' organism

2.1 The influence of phytobiotics on growth and performance of broiler chickens

The use of plant additives in poultry rearing can improve the absorption, use and absorption of valuable nutrients, and also stimulate the immune system. Phytogenic feed additives very often improve palatability and feed conversion, which in turn can lead to improved efficiency of poultry rearing (body weight, feed

Plant	Used part/ material	Active component	Beneficial effect	References
Cinnamon (*Cinnamomum zeylanicum*)	bark, leaves/ cinnamon oil	cinnamaldehyde eugenol, phenolic and polyphenolic substances	improves of appetite and digestion; enhances of antioxidant status; actions antimicrobial and blood purifying; alleviation of adverse effect of environmental stress; chemopreventive effect	[6, 10–12]
Garlic (*Allium sativum*)	crushed bulbs	allicin, ajoene, allyldisulfide, vinyldithiin, phytosterols, mucilages, pectins, flavonoids	improves immunity by increasing the titer of antibodies, stimulating the activity of lysozyme and increases the phagocytic activity of macrophages; chemopreventive effect, actions antiseptic and alleviate adverse effect of environmental stress; improves of digestion and the blood lipid profile; improve of growth and FCR	[11, 13–16]
Coneflower (*Echinacea purpurea*)	leaves root/ dried herb, water and alcohol extracts, root	polysaccharides, flavonoids, polyphenolic acids - mainly chlorogenic acid and caffeic acid, alkylamides, polyacetylenes	immunomodulatory - stimulates phagocytic activity of macrophages, increases the activity of lysozyme, increases the titer of antibodies; antimicrobial, antitumor, antidiabetic, and antioxidant, digestion stimulant, improves of growth and FCR	[6, 8, 14, 17–22]
Moringa (*Moringa oleifera*)	leaves/ extracts	chlorogenic acid, caffeicacid, ascorbic acid, flavonoids, phenolics and carotenoids	improves in egg production and decreases FCR; alleviates adverse effect of environmental stress; improves in egg production and decreases FCR; alleviates adverse effect of environmental stress; antioxidant activity	[2, 10, 23–25]
Pappermint (*Mentha piperita*)	leaves/ powder	menthol, terpenes	enhances of appetite and stimulate of digestion; causes decrease of FCR; it works antiseptic; improves in the laying performance, quality and freshness of eggs, and an color or the chemical composition of yolk	[14, 23, 26–28]

Plant	Used part/ material	Active component	Beneficial effect	References
Turmeric (*Curcuma longa*)	rhizome/ powder	curcuminoids, turmerones,	improves the blood lipid profile; improves digestion - choleretic, increases appetite; action antioxidative; anticarcinogenic; antihepatotoxic and immunomodulatory - stimulates the production of interferon; chemopreventive effect	[29, 30]
Aloe vera (*Aloe barbadensis*)	leaves/water extracts, powder, gel powder	anthraquinones polisaccharides (mainly icemannan) vitamins, enzymes, salicylic acid, anthraquinones and lignin, aminoacids	immunomodulation - stimulates the activity of granulocytes and granulocytic enzymes (myeloperoxidase, peroxidase), increases the titer of antibodies; alleviate adverse effect of environmental stress; action antidiabetic, and antioxidant - decreasing the lipid peroxidation and increasing the antioxidant status; stimulation of digestion - improve absorption of nutrients from the intestine, improve of intestinal microflora; improve of performance and FCR; increasing and providing protection to the vital phisiological organ like liver and kidney	[29–33]
Ginger (*Zingiber officinale*)	roots/ extracted basic oil	monoterpenes and sesquiterpenes	improves body weight gain due to stimulation of digestive enzymes and improvement of overall digestion, inhibits the growth of harmful bacteria in the intestinal tract due to antimicrobial activity lead to assimilation of nutrients, improves carcass traits, decreases abdominal fat; immunomodulation - increases the activity of lysozyme; chemopreventive effect	[28]

Table 1.
Effect of different herbs on the physiological functions and performance of poultry.

consumption, feed conversion, daily weight gain, mortality, etc.) (**Table 1**) [34]. According to Wenk et al. [13], dietary plant extracts strongly stimulate the endocrine system and indirect metabolism of nutrients. Many plant additives, including cinnamon, ginger, garlic, fenugreek, oregano, ribwort plantain, thyme, sage, marjoram, echinacea, lemon balm, cumin, peppermint, nettle, chamomile, sea buckthorn, milk thistle whether alfalfa, can stimulate metabolism and the absorption of nutrients, prevent inflammation of the digestive tract, has a tonic effect, prevent diarrhea, improve intestinal immunity and the composition of the microbiome (by competing with pathogens, the gut microbiome increase enterocytes permeability and nutrient absorption, and creates a protective biofilm that limits or inhibits the colonization and multiplication of pathogenic bacteria), has antiparasitic, anti-inflammatory and antioxidant properties, which in turn improve the birds' health. The effect of limiting the multiplication and adhesion of pathogens is the improvement of the structure and functioning of enterocytes, as well as acceleration of the maturation of cells of the intestinal immune system and strengthening of the immune response [14].

Moreover, the addition of phytobiotics increases the secretion and activity of digestive enzymes and the speed of digestion, stimulates the work of the pancreas and liver [35]. According to Rao et al. [36] Lee et al. [37] and Jang [38], essential oils and plant extracts administered in the feed of broilers, stimulate the secretion of amylase, maltase, trypsin and pancreatic lipase. Additive 100 ppm and 200 ppm essential oil derived from cinnamon do diet of chickens causes an improvement in the live weight gain and the health of broilers and feed conversion ratio (FCR) [10]. The addition of garlic or turmeric powder at 0.5% to the chickens' diet, can improve of broiler growth and feed conversion ratio (FCR) and decreased mortality rate [11, 15]. The improvement in yield may be related to the presence of various important alkaloids that have a positive effect on the health of broilers. For example, the sanguinarine is an alkaloid with excellent biological properties [17], positively influencing gastric motility, fermentation process and intestinal histomorphology [18]. Hernandez et al. [19] showed that the supplementation of diet by Rosmarinus officinal is, carvacrol, cinnamonaldehyde and capsaicin can improve feed digestibility in broilers. Aroche et al. [2] suggested that polyphenols, and especially tannins obtained from the leaves of *A. occidentale*, have the ability can bind to saliva lubricating proteins by hydrogen bonds; therefore, an increase of this metabolite in the diet could reduce the passage of the digesta in the gastro-intestinal tract and decrease the feed intake by a higher state of satiety in this period. However, an excess of tannins can provoke metabolic disturbances leading to an antinutritional influence, such as inhibiting the absorption of iron and sulfur containing amino acids causing anemia and depression of growth. The addition of calendula or corn to the diet improves the color of the broiler carcass, giving the skin a yellow tint. The addition of mint and pansy to the chickens diet increases the proportion of unsaturated acids change the fatty acid profile in the meat, while hops, nettle and lemon adversely change the fatty acid profile in meat, increasing the proportion of polyunsaturated fats [20]. Al-Kassie [10]; El-Ghousein et al. [21]; and Najafi et al., [22] showed a very beneficial effect of thyme on the efficiency of poultry rearing also. The addition of phytobiotics to water or feed also improves egg production, chemical composition and egg quality. For example, ginger essential oil or powder ginger (100–150 μl/kg body weight), when applied to water or poultry feed, can improve improves laying performance, chemical composition and egg quality. The use of plant additives in poultry rearing may contribute to increasing the weight of eggs and the thickness and strength of their shells, as well as stimulating the laying rate and contributing to the extension of the laying period [8, 39, 40]. The addition of garlic powder (1–5%), ginger, mulberry, black cumin, black seed, thyme, mentha and goldthread to the diet of laying hens increases the weight of the egg, the protein content of the egg and egg yolk antioxidants contain [9, 28, 41–46]. Swain et al. [47] observed that the addition of moringa leaf flour to the diet of chickens (5 g/kg) can also increases egg production (increases the number of eggs laid and improves their consumption quality). An important advantage of using phytobiotics in egg production is also the can improve egg quality and the vitelline membrane integrity besides enhancing antibody titer against Newcastle disease, as well as the color of the yolk and the quality of the protein, and eggs' freshness [42, 48, 49]. In practice, a factor contributing to increasing the yolk color intensity in a slow-ranging system is supplementing the diet with plants that are a source of xanthophylls, especially lutein, present in pumpkin, marigold, corn kernels, parsley or chives [40, 42, 50]. Supplementing the diet with plant ingredients or biologically active substances of herbs can improve the nutritional value of table eggs. Often, using phytobiotics in the diet of laying hens can reduces the amount of cholesterol in the yolk, the excess of which in the diet promotes the development of atherosclerosis in humans and stimulates the development of harmful free radical reactions in blood vessels. To reduce cholesterol in the yolk worth applying addition of garlic, ginger, black cumin, black seed, nettle, black tea, sage, thyme and mentha [43, 44, 51–53]. For this purpose, eggs are enriched with polyunsaturated fatty acids, and the oxidative stability of the yolk's lipids is improved. Using of ginger in layer diets can also advantageously increase activity of antioxidants enzymes and decreased content of MDA (harmful product of lipid peroxidation) and cholesterol in yolk [28, 54, 55]. Swain et al. [47] observed that additive of moringa leaf meal to chicken diet (5 g/kg) causes decrease of feed conversion ratio (FCR). Cayan et al. [55] observed that olive leaf powder added to chicken diet can increase yellowness in yolk color and decrease of yolk cholesterol content about 10%. Sunder et al. [56] showed that daily consumption of Indian mulberry (*Morinda citrifolia*) powder by hens increases the egg weight and the thickness of the egg shell. According to Cayan et al. [55] supplementation of the diet of laying hens with 0.1 and 0.5% the addition of thyme, improves feed conversion and egg production. Santoso et al. [57] reported that supplementation 5% addition of papaya leaf extract can improve body weight gain and carcass quality in broiler chickens, and increase egg protein content. The scientific literature contains also numerous reports indicating that phytobiotics do not significantly affect growth performance, feed conversion ratio and the survival rate of poultry but regulate the physiological functions of the organism (metabolism, activity of important enzymes, the level of minerals or blood composition) [5, 58, 59].

2.2 Influence of phytobiotics on the course of physiological reactions

Phytobiotic additives allow to regulate the course of physiological reactions, often conditioned by the activity of appropriate enzymes and hormones, at the level of metabolic biochemical changes in cells [5, 59, 60]. Plant additives can also improve the course of physiological functions, thus improving the performance of birds (**Table 2**) [14]. The use of e.g. cinnamon oil, garlic, echinacea, narrow-leaved

Plant	Used part/ material	Active component	Beneficial effect	References
Cinnamon (*Cinnamomum zeylanicum*)	bark, leaves/ cinnamon oil	cinnamaldehyde, eugenol, phenolic and polyphenolic substances	increase the proportion of HDL cholesterol, reduction of total cholesterol and triacylglycerols level, decrease lactate dehydrogenase, creatine kinase and β-hydroxybutyrate dehydrogenase activity, normalize the activity of aminotransferases	[6, 8, 10, 61]
Garlic (*Allium sativum*)	crushed bulbs	allicin, ajoene, allyldisulfide, vinyldithiin, phytosterols, mucilages, pectins, flavonoids	increase of HDL content, decrease of total cholesterol and triacylglycerols level,	[60]
Coneflower (*Echinacea purpurea*)	leaves root/ dried herb, water and alcohol extracts	polysaccharides, flavonoids, polyphenolic acids - mainly chlorogenic acid and caffeic acid, alkylamides, polyacetylenes	increase of HDL content, decrease of total cholesterol and triacylglycerols level	[59]

Plant	Used part/ material	Active component	Beneficial effect	References
Lavender (*Lavandula angustifolia*)	the whole plant, oil	hydrocarbons, alcohols, ketones, esters, aldehydes, oxides, and ethers coumarins and organic acids	beneficially effects on lipids' digestion and absorption due enhance the synthesis and excretion of bile acids in the liver, it could improve the lipids' digestion and absorption, decrease of total cholesterol	[6]
Pappermint (*Mentha piperita*)	leaves/powder	menthol, terpenes	decrease of total cholesterol, triacylglycerols, LDL and glucose level, increase of HDL level,	[14, 26, 27, 62]
Nettle (*Urtica dioica*)	leaves, root/ water extracts	organic acids carotenoids flavonoids tannins organic compounds, phytoestrogens, sterols, fatty acids	improves serum lipid profile, decrease of triglycerides and total cholesterol in the blood;	[51]
Ginger (*Zingiber officinale*)	roots/ extracted basic oil	monoterpenes and sesquiterpenes	improves serum lipid profile, decreases of triglycerides and total cholesterol serum features, total protein, globulin and antioxidant enzymes were elevated	[28]
Oregano (*Origanum vulgare*)	leaves/oil	terpenoids: carvacrol and thymol, polyphenols	increase of HDL content, decrease of total cholesterol and triacylglycerols level, oxidative stability of the produced meat	[63]
Shinyprivet (*Ligustrum lucidum*)	bark, twigs, flowers / water decoctions	nuzenide, oleuropein, oleanolic acid, betulin	decrease levels of cholesterol, LDL cholesterol, triglycerides and alanine aminotransferase activity, increased blood serum level of HDL	[64]

Table 2.
Effect of different herbs on the biochemical components of poultry blood.

lavender, mint, nettle, ginger, oregano and shiny privet in the diet of chickens can to reduce the level of triacylglycerols in the blood, increase the proportion of HDL cholesterol (due to inhibition of 3-hydroxy-3-methylglutaryl reductase coenzyme A, a key enzyme in the synthesis of cholesterol), and also favorably reduce or normalize the activity of aminotransferases [6, 8, 51, 59, 60, 64, 65], as well as lactate dehydrogenase, creatine kinase and β-hydroxybutyrate dehydrogenase [6].

Moreover, Krauze et al. [6] thinking, that the increase in NEFA levels in the blood of chickens suggests a very beneficial, inhibitory effect of cinnamon oil on the synthesis of triacylglycerols, due to the use of glycerol for glucose synthesis in the process of gluconeogenesis [66]. Of course, there are many examples of the use of plant additives that stimulate physiological reactions in the world literature. Fenita et al. [67] declared that adding a 3% addition of noni powder to feed can lower cholesterol and triglycerides in the blood of chickens, even below 50%. The research concerns various doses, forms and frequency of use, both extracts and dried material, or extracted biologically active substances, administered with feed or drinking water. It is also important to add that other forms of plant additives also, which have recently become very popular, are used for this purpose, i.e. fermented products, e.g. from soybean or rapeseed, improving the metabolic profile of poultry [68, 69]. Research has shown that herbal supplements can also reduce stress in poultry. Maryati et al. [70] and Muthmainnah et al. [71] believe that a 5% addition of essential oil from basil leaves to chickens improves the hematological profile of their blood. Such an additive can be, for example, aloe, which, by reducing the level of corticosterone in the blood, reduces the organism's susceptibility to stress factors and improves bird welfare. Moreover, the addition of sage, nettle or lemon to the diet of chickens reduces the stress response before slaughter [72].

2.3 Antimicrobial influence of phytobiotics and their influence on intestinal morphometry

Among the many plant additives the strongest antibacterial and antifungal properties can oils and plant extracts of thyme, echinacea, oregano, sage, garlic and cinnamon, rich in polyphenols. [72, 73]. The antimicrobial action of plant bioactive substances (polyphenols, especially flavonoids; and also tannins, coumarins, triterpenoids, isoprene derivatives, glucosinolates and alkaloids) is based on the disintegration of pathogen cell membrane structures what causing the migration of valuable ions from the pathogen's cell to the external environment, thus reducing their virulence [34, 74]. Research by Pasqua et al. [75] it have shown that limonene or cinnamic aldehyde can even destroy the structure of long-chain fatty acids in the cell membranes of *E. coli* bacteria. It has been suggested that the hydrophobicity of essential oils plays a key role in promoting the penetration of the phospholipid layer of the mitochondrial and cellular membrane of bacteria, leading to leakage of critical cell components and ions leading to cell death of these pathogens [76]. According to Castillo et al. [77] phytobiotics have a probiotic effect, and by selectively regulating the composition of the intestinal microbiota, they help maintain the eubiosis state [73, 77]. The results of the research conducted by the research team represented by Castillo et al. [77] showed, that a mixture of cinnamaldehyde, capsaicin and carvacrol stimulates the increase in the number of lactobacilli in the gastrointestinal tract. On the other hand, the results of the research by Jamroz [78] indicate that the herbal extract containing 5% carvacrol, 3% cinnamaldehyde and 2% capsicum oleoresin causes the formation of a thick layer of mucus on the chickens' stomach wall and jejunum. The formation of such a film reduces the possibility of the adherence of pathogens to the intestinal epithelium, which reduces the number of *Escherichia coli* and *Clostridium perfringens* bacteria and fungi in the intestines of birds. Stabilization of the intestinal microflora is particularly important in the critical periods of the animal production cycle, characterized by high susceptibility to health disorders, e.g. during chick rearing, change type of food, which is related to the age of birds, or, for example, the creating corals in turkeys. The addition of phytobiotics makes the birds less vulnerable to bacteria, toxins and other unwanted bacterial metabolites, such as ammonia and biogenic amines [79]. According to Puvača et al. [80] a significant number of bioactive substances present in essential oils leads to a reduction of the *Clostridium sp*. population in the digestive tract and poultry feces. Recently, high hopes have been associated with the use of preparations based on cinnamon, e.g. bark, powder or oil, containing cinnamic acid or aldehyde, stimulating the growth of lactobacilli in the gastrointestinal tract. Cayan et al. [55] suggested that supplementation diet of laying hens with 0.1 and 0.5%, the addition of thyme reduces the content of *E. colifecal*. The results of the research [6] showed that the use of a commercial preparation containing cinnamon oil (0.25 mL/L of drinking water) is able to improve the microbiome and morphometry of the small intestine of broiler chickens. Interesting results of research on the administration of plant additives were presented by Maryati et al. [70] and

Muthmainnah et al. [71] who showed that a 5% addition of essential oil from basil leaves administered to the feed can have antibacterial activity against *S. aureus* and *E. coli*. This oil owes its antibacterial properties to hydrocarbons, alcohols, esters, phenols (contains 1–19% of eugenol, iso-eugenol), phenolic ether (contains 3–31% methyl clavicol, 1–9% methyl eugenol), numerous oxides and ketones. Another valuable plant additive administered with the feed that reduces the production of toxic ammonia in the digestive tract of chickens is *Yucca schidigera* extract, which contains numerous saponins. Nazeer et al. [81] claims that such an addition significantly reduces the activity of urease in the intestines and feces in broilers fed with such an extract. It should be emphasized that the advantage of herbs is the selectivity of their antibacterial action, which will not be observed when using antibiotics. The antibiotic limits the multiplication of both harmful and beneficial bacteria, while the herbal extract used, for example, from cinnamon, thyme and oregano, only limits the growth of pathogenic bacteria. It should be noted, however, that such an effect is achieved with highly concentrated herbal extracts containing a mixture of various bioactive substances [79].

2.4 The influence of plant additives on bird immunity

From plant additives, stimulating the immune system, it is expected to improve the immune status, and consequently to streng then, the immunity of animals, improve their health and productivity. Plant preparations administered in the diet can increase the phagocytic activity of macrophages, increase the titer of antibodies and stimulated B and T lymphocytes, increase the level of lysozyme, stimulate the synthesis of interferon or have a chemopreventive effect (see **Table 1**). Herbs that stimulate the immune system include, among others: garlic, Echinacea, cinnamon, plantain, aloe, arnica, oregano, nettle and ginseng. The substances with a strong immunostimulatory effect are mainly: polyphenols, sulfur compounds, alkaloids, terpenes, saponins, essential oils and tannins [82]. The main components of valuable essential oils are lipophilic, liquid and volatile components, i.e. alcohols, aldehydes, esters, ethers, ketones, phenols and terpenes [83]. According to Aroche et al. [2], inclusion of mixed powder with *Anacardium occidentale* (60%), *Psidium guajava* (20%), and *Morinda citrifolia* (20%) to chicken diet can help with a quick immune system response and to improve immunity. This supplement exerts a beneficial immune effect, through an increase in the immunoglobulin G (IgG) concentration and with a synthesis of appropriate immune cells (macrophages). An increased immunoglobulin concentration has been associated with a benefit in the immune status, and IgG (with IgA) are the main immunoglobulins protecting against pathogenic microorganisms, mainly to intestinal level. IgG is one of the main defense barriers during the bacterial attack in the gastrointestinal tract (GIT), and the early proliferation of this cell is essential to improve the feed efficiency in these animals. The level of serum antibodies is an important indicator to know the effect of a natural product on immune response in animals [2]. Similar opinion has Tajodini et al. [84] who using artichoke powder (*Cynara scolymus*) in the diet of broilers found that this product significantly increased serum antibodies, resulting in a higher activity of the immune system. The results of the research [6] showed that the use of a preparation containing cinnamon oil (0.25 mL/L of drinking water) could improve the metabolism, and on the chickens' immunity.

2.5 Antioxidant effect of phytogenic substances

The health-promoting effect of plant antioxidants results from their protective counteracting both during the formation and the impact of reactive oxygen species. The results of the research showed that the antioxidant activity of herbs reduces the risk of cancer, heart disease, hypertension and stroke; and in the case of food of animal origin, it can minimize the rancidity process, delay the formation of toxic oxidation in products and keeps maintain the nutritional quality of the product [85]. Oxidation processes that generate free radicals, take place in the organism of animals in a continuous manner. Nevertheless, they are counterbalanced by complex antioxidant mechanism (enzymatic and non-enzymatic antioxidants) that minimize the toxic effects of the effects of reactive oxygen species (ROS). ROS are responsible for damaging lipids, proteins and DNA, as well as for disrupting immune defense. This may lead to qualitative changes in animal tissues, reducing their health, as well as lowering the quality of animal products (meat, milk, eggs), and also shortening their shelf life [72]. Antioxidant properties have polyphenols, especially flavonoids, tannins, phenols, terpenes and hydrolysable proanthocyanins, which are responsible for maintaining the correct level of glutathione in cells and for the protection of membrane lipids against peroxidation. Among the flavonoids, hesperidin, diosmin, dolphinin, epicatechin, resveratrol, kaempferol, quercetin and luteolin, which are particularly rich in citrus fruits and grapes, have the strongest antioxidant properties [85]. According to Caillet et al. [86], these compounds can inhibit the formation of ROS and form stable complexes (so-called chelates) with transition metals (Cu^{2+} and Fe^{2+}), thus preventing Fenton and Haber-Weiss reactions. Flavonoids break the cascade of free radical reactions (capturing lipid and alkoxy free radicals) leading to lipid peroxidation, thus protecting other antioxidants (especially cytosolic ascorbate and biological membranes tocopherol). The group of herbs with antioxidant properties includes many plants [87] but the strongest antioxidant potential is shown by cloves (total antioxidants: 125.50–465.32 mmol/100 g), oregano (total antioxidants: 96.64–137.50 mmol/100 g), marjoram (total antioxidants: 55.80–92.31 mmol/100 g) and sage (total antioxidants: 34.88–91.20 mmol/100 g) [88, 89]. The antioxidant effect of herbs is manifested through modification of the activity of antioxidant enzymes, increasing the total antioxidant potential blood plasma (FRAP) or its components, as well as by protecting lipids against the peroxidation process, consisting in oxidative damage to the structures of lipid components of tissues and decreasing level of oxidation products, especially lipids (especially malondialdehyde, dienes and lipid hydroperoxides) [87]. Studies have shown that in the case of poultry rearing, rosemary, oregano, calendula, sage, cloves, garlic, ginger and saffron are primarily used, preventing the lipid oxidation processes in meat [90, 91] and in eggs [92]. Shirzadegan [93] found that supplementing the diet of chickens with a mixture containing green tea extract, cinnamon, garlic and chicory in the proportion of 25:15:45:14 in the amount of 2,5; 5,0 and 7,5 g/kg of feed improves antioxidant status and hepatic superoxide dismutase activity, which protects hepatocytes from the harmful effects of lipid peroxidation. The results of the research [6] on chicken showed that the use of a preparation containing cinnamon oil (0,25 mL/L of drinking water) increased of anti-oxidants level in the blood. Faix et al. [94] also states that the components of cinnamon oil increase the activity of antioxidant enzymes, thereby inhibiting lipid peroxidation. Lambert et al. [95] suggests that some plant additives, especially in an inappropriate dose, may show a pro-oxidative effect, intensifying the oxidation reactions in the system and in the food. Plant components with such characteristics include coriander, cardamom, verbena, sage, eucalyptus, lemon, and tarragon.

2.6 The harmful and toxic plants for poultry

In free-range breeding, poultry loves to roam the garden and treat all plants, especially garden flowers (e.g. marigolds), flowers and fruits of pumpkins and zucchini, and weeds, e.g. dandelions, as potential food. Of course, abundant supplies of fresh fruit, vegetables and garden greens are part of their balanced diet, but not all garden plants are good for breeding birds. In fact, some are toxic and many biologically active plant compounds can cause poisoning, disease and even death. The possibility of consumption of toxic plants by birds exposes potential consumers of animal products to poisoning, due to the fact that toxic substances easily penetrate into meat or eggs. World centers dealing with the issues of plant toxicity to livestock publish lists of plants classified according to the degree of toxicity, sensitivity of individual animal species, or according to the content of toxins [96]. The main potentially toxic compounds are alkaloids, mainly purine and quinoline, occurring in plants in the form of salts of organic acids [97, 98]. They contain heterocyclic systems with an oxygen or nitrogen atom in their molecule and are basic in nature. Such compounds are present p. e. in coffee, tea, monkshood and poppy seeds. The next ones are glycosides, which give the plant a characteristic taste and smell (e.g. amygdalin) or color (flavones, anthocyanins). Some of them have a bacteriostatic effect (sinigrin present in horseradish). The protein - myosin, can cause reproductive disorders, such as loss of coat or feathers [99]. On the other hand, aminopropionitrile, present in the lupine, contributes to the deformation of the skeleton, especially the long bones and the chest. Essential oils, aromatic oils in the form of colorless liquids can also be toxic. The chemical composition of these forms of plant additives is often very diverse (aliphatic and aromatic compounds, terpenes, alcohols, phenols, hydrocarbons, aldehydes, ketones and esters). Resins, which are a mixture of organic acids, alcohols, phenols, esters and carbohydrates, or photosensitizing compounds (photosensitizing) are also dangerous for animals. Insoluble calcium oxalates can take the form of kidney stones in the kidneys, and their genesis comes from the oxalic acid found in many vegetables and grasses [97–100]. The content of potentially toxic substances is also influenced by the climate, soil type, companionship of other plants, as well as the method of storage and processing. Often the forage may be contaminated with toxic weed kernels. The seeds of *Senna occidentalis* (formerly called *Cassia occidentalis*) are among such dangers. The entire plant is toxic, but the most toxic, is dianthrone (anthraquinone derivative) has been identified in the outer and inner shells. It turned out that this substance can cause the characteristic mitochondrial myopathy with impaired mitochondrial function, damage to the biological membrane and swelling of this organelle, leakage of the mitochondrial matrix, and disintegration of mitochondrial combs [101]. The results of the research by Gotardo et al. [102] showed that the toxic dianthrone caused damage to the ovaries in laying hens, yolk leakage around the hair follicles, probably due to an increase in the fragility and permeability of the vitelline membrane itself. This membrane is a protein extracellular matrix surrounding the oocyte filled with yolk, and by preventing the yolk from mixing with the protein, it constitutes a kind of barrier to microbial infection [103]. The inner layer of the vitelline membrane is synthesized in the ovary, prior to ovulation, in the form of a three-dimensional network of thick glycoprotein fibrils. Assuming that the metabolic energy cost of follicle development and egg production in laying hens is high, and the toxic dianthrone damages the structure and function of mitochondria and leads to depletion of glycogen energy reserves, losses can be significant [104, 105]. If we take into account that anthraquinone affects mitochondrial functions, leading to glycogen depletion in cells, it can be assumed that the direct action of this compound in the ovary would lead to lower energy production in this organ, and consequently affect egg formation, possibly due to an increase in the fragility and/or permeability of the vitelline membrane. It is well known that toxins such as aflatoxin and the alkaloid pyrrolizidine plants can endanger egg production too [106]. The following plants are particularly dangerous for poultry:

yew, rhubarb, periwinkle, oak teres, nightshades, lupine, lobelia, holly, foxglove, ferns, bulbs of garden plants, beans, azalia and apricots. The acorns, that fall from oaks in autumn, contain tannic acid, which can cause a lack of appetite and diarrhea [107]. Dangerous oxalates can be found in rhubarb, sorrel and spinach; but cut twigs, fallen needles, and yew berries containing cardiotoxic taxin alkaloids can also cause poisoning. While oxalates interfere with kidney function, yew taxols cause cardiac arrhythmias and even lead to death [108]. Nightshades plants (i.e. tomatoes, peppers, eggplant, bittersweet and Jerusalem cherry, potatoes) can be harmful to poultry. Nightshades plants contain glycoalkaloids that cause loss of appetite, increased salivation, reduced heart rate and difficulty breathing. Growers should pay particular attention to raw potato skins, which are particularly dangerous to poultry. Lupine contains quinolizidine alkaloids, which may deteriorate the nutritional and organoleptic quality of poultry meat, and cause nervousness, depression, muscle tremors and convulsions in birds [109]. Lobelia contains toxins belonging to the pyridine alkaloids that can cause neurological changes, weakness, faster breathing and lack of motor coordination in poultry. The shiny green leaves and red berries of holly have a low level of toxicity, however the leaves contain highly poisonous saponins that can cause red blood cell damage, vomiting, diarrhea and drooling in chickens [110]. All parts of the beautiful foxglove (seeds, flowers, stems and leaves), who produces bright tubular flowers with mottled insides, are toxic [111, 112]. A specific variety of fern called the "bracken fern" can cause poisoning in chickens, weight loss and muscle tremorswhich, and to lead to anemia. Many varieties of garden plant bulbs (daffodils, irises, narcissi, tulips) contain highly toxic alkaloids that lower blood pressure and disrupt the heart, causing neurological changes and causing diarrhea. Raw beans contain haemagglutinins that are highly toxic to chickens, damaging and clumping blood erythrocytes [99, 112]. In azaleas, all parts of the plant are highly toxic and can cause digestive disorders, weakness, neurological disorders and loss of motor coordination, as well as damage to cardiomyocytes. Apricot leaves and kernels contain highly toxic cyanogenic glycosides, which cause symptoms such as seizures, breathing problems and low blood pressure. When leaves are exposed to frost, drought or disease, the level of toxicity increases [111, 112]. Due to the potential toxicity of some herbs, and the use of incorrect doses (too large doses) of herbs with a potentially beneficial effect, it is definitely more advantageous to use ready-made, standardized phytobiotic additives for poultry, where the manufacturer precisely specifies a safe and effective dose of the preparation with a standardized amount of active substances.

3. Conclusion

Summarizing the impact of phytobiotics used in poultry rearing, it can be noted that these additives:

1. improve growth and performance of broiler chickens, through greatly improve digestion and nutrient assimilation, and modify the composition of the intestinal microbiota and improve intestinal morphometry.

2. stimulate physiological reactions, especially immunity, but they also favorably modify the blood lipid profile, increase the antioxidant defense of the body, as well as increase resistance to stress.

3. they improve the quality of meat and eggs, increase the weight of valuable parts of carcass (pectoral and leg muscles) and stimulate laying.

4. due to the potentially toxic effect of an excess of certain herbs on the work of the liver, and the adverse changes in the palatability of eggs, use caution in the use some herbs e.g. of garlic, turmeric, rapeseed, alfa alfa, shiny privet or moringa.

4. Conclusions for practice

Due to the health-promoting properties of herbs and plant preparations, it is worth using such supplements in practice, because in this way you can increase the effects of chicken rearing and improve the quality of meat and eggs. The best results can be obtained by using proven and well-known plant additives, especially cinnamon, ginger, coneflower, nettle or aloe. Increasing the intensity of the yolk color desired by egg consumers can be obtained by feeding the laying hens with calendula, pumpkin, chives or parsley.

In large poultry farms, the easiest solution is to use ready-made plants' preparations to drinking water or feed.

Conflict of interest

The authors declare no conflict of interest.

Author details

Magdalena Krauze
Department of Biochemistry and Toxicology, Faculty of Animal Sciences and Bioeconomy, University of Life Sciences in Lublin, Lublin, Poland

*Address all correspondence to: magdalena.krauze@up.lublin.pl

References

[1] Jarić S, Popović Z, Macukanović-Jocić M, Djurdjević L, Mijatović M, Karadzić B, Mitrović M, Pavlović P: An ethnobotanical study on the usage of wild medicinal herbs from Kopaonik Mountain (Central Serbia). Journal Ethnopharmacology. 2007;20:160-175. DOI: 10.1016/j.jep.2006.11.007.

[2] Aroche R, Martínez Y, Ruan Z, Guan G, Waititu S, Nyachoti CM: Dietary inclusion of a mixed powder of medicinal plant leaves enhances the feed efficiency and immune function in broiler chickens. Journal of Chemistry 2018;394:1-6.doi.org/10.1590/1806-9061-2020-1362.

[3] Jakhetia V, Patel R, Khatri P: Cinnamon: A pharmacological review. Journal of Advanced Scientific Research. 2010;1:19-23.

[4] Sang-Oh P, Chae-Min R, Byung-Sung P. Jong H: The meat quality and growth performance in broiler chickens fed diet with cinnamon powder. Journal of Environmental Biology. 2013;34:127-133.

[5] Krauze M, Grela ER: Effects of an alfalfa concentrate in Turkey diets on performance and some blood parameters. Archiv für Geflugelkunde. 2010;74:226-232.

[6] Krauze M, Cendrowska-Pinkosz M, Matusevicius P, Stępniowska A, Jurczak P, Ognik K: The effect of administration of a phytobiotic containing cinnamon oil and citric acid on the metabolism, immunity, and growth performance of broiler chickens. Animals. 2021;11:399. DOI.org/10.3390/ani11020399.

[7] Alagawany M, Elnesr SS, Farag MR: Use of liquorice (*Glycyrrhiza glabra*) in poultry nutrition: Global impacts on performance, carcass and meat quality. World's Poultry Science Journal. 2019;75: 293-304. DOI.org/10.1017/S0043933919000059.

[8] Abd El-Hack ME, Alagawany M, Abdel-Moneim AME, Mohammed NG, Khafaga AF, Bin-Jumah M, Othman SI, Allam AA, Elnesr SS: Cinnamon (Cinnamomum zeylanicum) oil as a potential alternative to antibiotics in poultry. Antibiotics. 2020a;9:210.

[9] Abd El-Hack A, Mohamed E, Alagawany M, Shaheen H, Samak D, Othman SI, Allam A, Taha A, Khafaga AF, Osman A: Ginger and its derivatives as promising alternatives to antibiotics in poultry feed. Animals. 2020b;10:452.

[10] Al-Kassie GA: Influence of two plant extracts derived from thyme and cinnamon on broiler performance. Pakistan Veterinary Journal. 2009; 29:169-173.DOI:10.1093/ps/83.2.169.

[11] Akyildiz S, Denli M: Application of plant extracts as feed additives in poultry nutrition. Animal Science. 2016;59:2285-5750.

[12] Chachaj R, Sembratowicz I, Krauze M, Stępniowska A, Rusinek-Prystupa E, Czech A, Matusevičius P, Ognik K: The effect of fermented soybean meal on performance, biochemical and immunological blood parameters in turkeys. Annals of Animal Science. 2019;19:1035-1049. doi: https://doi.org/10.2478/aoas-2019-0040.

[13] Wenk C. Herbs and botanicals as feed additives in monogastric animals. Asian-Australas Journal of Animal Science. 2003;16:282-289.

[14] Vinus RD, Sheoran N, Maan NS, Tewatia BS: Potential benefits of herbal supplements in poultry feed: A review. The Pharma Innovation Journal. 2018;7,651-656.

[15] Yarru LP, Settivari RS, Gowda NKS, Antoniou E, Ledoux DR, Rottinghaus GE: Effects of turmeric (Curcuma longa) on the expression of hepatic genes associated with biotransformation, antioxidant, and immune systems in broiler chicks fed aflatoxin. Poult Science. 2009;88: 2620-2262.

[16] Truchliński J, Krauze, Cendrowska-Pinkosz M, Modzelewska-Banachiewicz B: Influence of garlic, synthetic 1,2,4-triasole derivative and herbal preparation Echinovit C on selected indices of Turkey-hens non-specific immunity. Polish Journal of Veterinary Science. 2006;9:51-55.

[17] Abudabos AM, Alyemni AH, Dafalla YM, Khan RU: Effect of organic acid blend and Bacillus subtilis alone or in combination on growth traits, blood biochemical and antioxidant status in broiler exposed to Salmonella typhimurium challenge during the starter phase. Journal of Applied Animal Research. 2016;45:538-542.

[18] Jankowski J, Zduńczyk Z, Juśkiewicz J, Koz1owski K, Lecewicz a, Jeroch H: Gastrointestinal tract and metabolic response of broilers to diets with the Macleaya cordata alkaloid extract. Archiv für Geflugelkunde. 2009;73:9-5101.

[19] Hernandez F, Madrid J, Garcia V, Orengo J, Megias MD: Influence of tow plant extracts on broiler performance, digestibility, and digestive organ size. Poultry Science. 2004;83:169-174.

[20] Kapica M, Kwiecień M, Puzio I, Bieńko M, Radzki R, Pawłowska M: Effect of selected herbs on the activity of digestive enzymes in broiler chickens. Veterinary Medicine, 2006;9: 1048-1050.

[21] El-Ghousein SS, Al-Beitawi NA: The effect of feeding of crushed thyme (*Thymus valgaris* L.) on growth, blood constituents, gastrointestinal tract and carcass characteristics of broiler chickens. The Journal of Poultry Science 2009;46:100-104.

[22] Najafi P, Torki M: Performance, blood metabolites and immuno competaence of broiler chicks fed diets included essential oils of medicinal herbs. Journal of Animal and Veterinary Advances 2010;9:1164-1168.

[23] Leone A, Spada A, Battezzati A, Schiraldi A, Aristil J, Bertoli S: Cultivation, genetic, ethnopharmacology, phytochemistry and pharmacology of Moringa oleifera leaves: An overview. International Journal of Molecular Science. 2015;16,12791-12835.

[24] Ogbunugafor HA, Eeneh FU, Ozumba AN, Igwoezikpe MN, Okpuzor J, Igwilo IO, Adenekan SO, Onyekwelu OA: Physicochemical and antioxidant properties of *Moringa oleifera* seed oil. Pakistan Journal of Nutrition. 2011;10,409-414. 28.

[25] Sofidiya MO, Odukoya OA, Familoni OB, Inyaagha SI: Free radical scavenging activity of some Nigerian medicinal plant extracts. Pakistan Journal of Biological Science. 2006;9,1438-1441.

[26] Abdel-Wareth AAA, Kehraus S, Südekum KH: Peppermint and its respective active component in diets of broiler chickens: Growth performance, viability, economics, meat physicochemical properties, and carcass characteristics. Poult Science. 2019;1;3850-3859. doi: 10.3382/ps/pez099.

[27] Asadi N, Husseini SD, Tohidian MT: Performance of broilers supplemented with peppermint (*Mentha piperita* L.) powder. The Journal of Evidence Based Integrative Medicine. 2018;22, 703-706. doi:10.1177/2156587217700771.

[28] Abd El-Hack ME, Alagawany, M.; Shaheen, H.; Samak, D.; Othman, S.I.; Allam, A.A.; Taha, A.E.; Khafaga AF. Arif M, Osman A, El Sheikh AI, Elnesr SS, Sitohy M: Ginger and its derivatives as promising alternatives to antibiotics in poultry feed. Animals. 2020;10,452.https://doi.org/10.3390/ani10030452.

[29] Darabighane B, Nahashon SN: A review on effects of aloe vera as a feed additive in broiler chicken diets. Annals of Animal Science. 2014;143,491-500. https://doi.org/10.2478/aoas-2014-0026.

[30] Sinha S, Muzamil S, Ahmad B, Rehman MU, Quadri A: "Ameliorative effect of *Aloe vera* supplementation in poultry feed" Journal of Animal Research. 2017; 7,1,85-90. doi:10.5958/2277-940X.2017.00012.2.

[31] Amany A, Ebrahim SS, Elnesr MAA. Abdel-Mageed M, Aly MM: Nutritional significance of aloe vera (*Aloe barbadensis* miller) and its beneficial impact on poultry. World's Poultry Science Journal. 2020;76:4,803-4,814. DOI: 10.1080/00439339.2020.1830010.

[32] Taraneh JFK: A study on the effects of supplementing *Aloe vera* gel and garlic powder on immune response of broiler." Global Journal of Poultry Farming and Vaccination. 2016;4,6, 238-6,242.

[33] Tariq H, Raman Rao PV, Mondal BC, Malla BA. Effect of aloe vera (*Aloe barbadensis*) and clove (*Syzigium aromaticum*) supplementation on immune status, haematological and serum biochemical parameters of japanese quails. Indian Journal of Animal Nutrition. 2014;31,3,293-3,296.

[34] Windisch W, Schedle K, Plitzner C. Kroismayr A: Use of phytogenic products as feed additives for swine and poultry. Journal of Animal Science. 2008;86:140-148.

[35] Suresh D, Srinivasan K: Studies on the in vitro absorption of spice principles – Curcumin, capsaicin and piperine in rat intestines. Food Chemistry and Toxicology 2007;45:1437-1442.

[36] Rao RR, Platel K, Srinivasan K: In vitro influence of spices and spice-active principles on digestive enzymes of rat pancreas and small intestine. Nährung. 2003;47:408-412.

[37] Lee MK, Park YB, Moon SS, Bok SH, Kim DJ, Ha TY, Jeong TS, Jeong KS, Choi MS: Hypo cholesterolemic and antioxidant properties of 3-(4-hydroxyl) propanoic acid derivatives in high-cholesterol fed rats. Chemico-Biological Interactions. 2007;170:9-19. DOI:10.1016/j.cbi.2007.06.037.

[38] Yang Y, Zhao L, Shao Y, Liao X, Zhang L, Lu L, Luo X: Effects of dietary graded levels of cinnamon essential oil and its combination with bamboo leaf flavonoid on immune function, antioxidative ability and intestinal microbiota of broilers. Journal of Integrative Agriculture. 2019;1: 2123-2132. DOI:10.1016/S2095-3119(19)62566-9.

[39] Osman A, El-Araby GM, Taha H: Potential use as a bio-preservative from lupin protein hydrolysate generated by alcalase in food system. Journal Applied Biology and Biotechnology. 2016;4, 076-081.

[40] Sirri F, Iaffaldano N, Minelli G, Meluzzi A, Rosato MP, Franchini A: Comparative pigmentation efficiency of high dietary levels of apoester and marigold extract on quality traits of whole liquid egg of two strains of laying hens. Journal of Applied Poultry Research. 2007;16:429-437.

[41] Olobatoke RY, Mulugeta SD: Effect of dietary garlic powder on layer performance, fecal bacterial load, and

egg quality. Poultry Science. 2011;90:665-670.

[42] Hojati H, Hassanabadi A, Ahmadian F: Application of medicinal plants in poultry nutrition, Journal of Medicinal plants and by-product, 3(1), 2014;1-12, doi: 10.22092/jmpb.2014.108597.

[43] Azeke MA, Ekpo KE: Egg yolk cholesterol lowering effect of garlic and tea. Journal of Biological Sciences. 2009;8,2,456-2,460.

[44] Mahmoud KZ, Gharaibeh SM, Zakaria HA, Qatramiz AM: Garlic (*Allium sativum*) supplementation: influence on egg production, quality, and yolk cholesterol level in layer hens. Asian-Australasian Journal of Animal Sciences. 2010;l,23,1503 – 1509.

[45] Xu X, Hu Y, Xiao W, Huang J, He X, Wu J, Ryan E, Weir TL: Effects of fermented *Camilla sinensis*, Fuzhuan tea, on egg cholesterol and production performance in laying hens, Agriculture and Food Science. 2021;1, 006-010.

[46] Tahan M, Bayram I: Effect of utilization of black cumin (*Nigella sativa*) and parsley (*Petroselinum crispum*) in laying quail diets on egg yield, egg quality and hatchability. Archiva Zootechnica. 2012;15,2 ,23-2,28.

[47] Swain BK, Naik PK, Chakurkar EB, Singh NP: Effect of supplementation of Moringa oleifera leaf meal (MOLM) on the performance of Vanaraja laying hens. Indian Journal of Animal Science. 2017;87:353-355.

[48] An S, Liu G, Guo X, An Y, Wang R: Ginger extract enhances antioxidant ability and immunity of layers. Animal Nutrition. 2019; 5,407-409.

[49] Poudel N, Khanal DR: Effect of stinging nettle feeding on productivity and immune status in laying hens. Nepalese Veterinary Journal. 2011;30,51-58.

[50] Skřivan M, Englmaierová M, Skrivanová E, Bubancová I: Increase in lutein and zeaxanthin content in the eggs of hens fed marigold flower extract. Czech Journal of Animal Science. 2015;60:89-96.

[51] Moula N, Sadoudi A, Touazi L, Leroy P, Geda F: Effects of stinging nettle (Urtica dioica) powder on laying performance, egg quality, and serum biochemical parameters of Japanese quails. Animal Nutrition. 2019;5:410-415. doi:10.1016/j.aninu.2019.05.002.

[52] Kaya H, Macit M: Effect of inclusion of garlic (*Allium sativum*) powder at different levels and copper into diets of hens on performance, egg quality traits and yolk cholesterol content. Inter J Poultry Science. 2012;11,114-119.

[53] Bölükbaşi ŞC, Kaynar Ö, Erhan MK, Ürüthan H: Effect of feeding Nigella sativa oil on laying hen performance, cholesterol and some proteins ratio of egg yolk and *Escherichia coli* count in feces. Journal Archiv für Geflügelkunde. 2009;73,167-172.

[54] Zhao X, Yang ZB, Yang WR, Wang Y, Jiang, SZ, Zhang GG: Effects of ginger root (*Zingiber officinale*) on laying performance and antioxidant status of laying hens and on dietary oxidation stability. Poultry Science. 2011;90,1720-1727.

[55] Cayan H, Erener G: Effect of olive leaf (Olea europaea) powder on laying hens performance, egg quality and egg yolk cholesterol levels. Asian-Australian Journal of Animal Science. 2015; 28:538-543.

[56] Sunder J, Sujatha T, Kundu A: Effect of Morinda citrifolia in growth, production and immunomodulatory properties in livestock and poultry: A review. Journal of Experimental Biology

and Agricultural Sciences. 2016; 249-265.

[57] Santoso U, Fenita Y, Kususiyah Y, Bidura IG: Effect of fermented *Sauropus androgynus* leaves on meat composition, amino acid and fatty acid compositions in broiler chickens. Pakistan Journal of Nutrition. 2015;14:799-807.

[58] Awad A, Fahim H, El-Shhat AEG, Mahrose K, Shazly S: Dietary *Echinacea purpurea* administration enhanced egg laying performance, serum lipid profile, antioxidant status and semen quality in duck breeders during summer season. Journal of Animal and Physiology and Animal Nutrition. 2021;https://doi.org/10.1111/jpn.13488

[59] Ognik K, Krauze M: The potential for using enzymatic assays to assess the health of turkeys. World Poultry Science Journal. 2016a:72:535– 550, doi:10.1017/S0043933916000246.

[60] Hossain MA, Mostofa M, Alam MN, Awal MA, Rahman MM: Effects of garlic (Allium sativum) feed supplement on hemato-biochemical properties in broiler chickens with sub-clinical toxicity of lead. Research in Agriculture, Livestock and Fisheries. 2014;1:87-96.

[61] Ciftci M, Simsek UG, Yuce A, Yilmaz O, Dalkilic B: Effects of dietary antibiotic and cinnamon oil supplementation on antioxidant enzyme activities, cholesterol levels and fatty acid compositions of serum and meat in broiler chickens. Acta Veterinaria Brno. 2010;79,33-40.

[62] Sorour HK, Hosny RA, Elmasry DMA: Effect of peppermint oil and its microemulsion on necrotic enteritis in broiler chickens, Veterinary World. 2021;14,2,483-2,491.

[63] Zamora M, Durán Meléndez G, Antonio L, Hume ME, Silva Vázquez S, Ramón V: (2017). Performance, blood parameters, and carcass yield of broiler chickens supplemented with Mexican oregano oil. Revista Brasileira de Zootecnia,2017;46,6,515-520.https://doi.org/10.1590/s1806-92902017000600006.

[64] Li XL, He WL, Yang ML, Yan YM, Xue YH, Zhao ST: Effect of dietary supplementation of *Ligustrum lucidum* on performance, egg quality and blood biochemical parameters of Hy-Line Brown hens during the late laying period. Animal. 2017;11,899-1904, ttps://doi.org/10.1017/S1751731117000532.

[65] Torki M, Mohebbifar A, Mohammadi H: Effects of supplementing hen diet with *Lavandula angustifolia* and/or *Mentha spicata* essential oils on production performance, egg quality and blood variables of laying hens. Veterinary Medicine and Science. 2021;7:184-193. https://doi.org/10.1002/vms3.343.

[66] Verago JL, Grassi-Kassisse DM, Spadari-Bratfisch RC: Metabolic markers following beta-adrenoceptor agonist infusion in footshock-stressed rats. The Brazilian Journal of Medical and Biological Research. 2001;34:1197-1207.

[67] Fenita Y: The influence of noni fruit flour in the ration on the percentage of internal organs, cholesterol and triglyceride levels of broiler blood. Proceeding of Semirata Field in Agricultural Sciences, Western Region, Bengkulu University, Bengkulu, Indonesia, 2010;1060-1065.

[68] Drażbo A, Kozłowski K, Ognik K, Zaworska A, Jankowski J: 2019. The effect of raw and fermented rapeseed cake on growth performance, carcass traits, and breast meat quality in Turkey. Poultry Science. 2019;98:6161-6169.

[69] Sembratowicz I, Chachaj R, Krauze M, Ognik K: The effect of diet

with fermented soybean meal on blood metabolites and redox status of chickens. Annals of Animal Science, 2020;20:599-611.

[70] Maryati RS, Fauzia T, Rahayu T: Antibacterial activity test of *Ocimum basilicum* L. toward Staphylococcus aureus and Escherichia coli. Indonesian Journal of Chemical Research, 2007;8:30-38.

[71] Muthmainnah R, Rubiyanto D, Julianto TS: Formulation of liquid soap made from active basil oil as antibacterial and testing against Staphylococcus aureus. Indonesian Journal of Chemical Research. 2014;1:44-50.

[72] Burt S: Essential oils: Their antibacterial properties and potential applications in food–a review. International Journal of Food Microbiology. 2004;94:223-253.

[73] Si W, Gong J, Tsao R, Zhou T, Yu H, Poppe C, Johnson R, Du Z: Antimicrobial activity of essential oils and structurally related synthetic food additives towards selected pathogenic and beneficial gut bacteria. Journal of Applied Microbiology. 2006;100: 296-305.

[74] Krauze M, Abramowicz K, Ognik K: The effect of the addition of probiotic bacteria (Bacillus subtilis or *Enterococcus faecium*) or phytobiotic containing cinnamon oil to drinking water on the health and performance of broiler chickens. Annals of Animal Science. 2020;20:191-205. DOI.org/10.2478/ aoas-2019-0059.

[75] Pasqua RD, Hoskins N, Betts G, Mauriello G: Changes in membrane fatty acids composition of microbial cells induced by addiction of thymol, carvacrol, limonene, cinnamaldehyde, and eugenol in the growing media. Journal of Agriculture and Food Chemistry. 2006;4:2745-2749.

[76] Prabuseenivasan S, Jayakumar M, Ignacimuthu S: 2006. In vitro antibacterial activity of some plant essential oils. BMC Complement. Alternative Medicine. 2006;6:39.

[77] Castillo M, Martin-Orue SM, Roca M, Manzanilla EG, Badiola I, Perez JF, Gasa J: The response of gastrointestinal microbiota to albamycin, butyrate, and plant extracts in early weaned pigs. Journal Animal Science. 2006;84:2725-2734.

[78] Jamroz D, Wertelecki T, Houszka M, Kamel C: Influence of diet type on the inclusion of plant origin active substances on morphological and histochemical characteristics of the stomach and jejunum walls in chicken. Journal of Animals Physiology and Animal Nutrition. 2006;90:255-268.

[79] Tipu MA, Akhtar MS, Anjum MI, Raja ML: New dimension of medicinal plants as animal feed. Pakistan Veterinary Journal. 2006;26:144-148.

[80] Puvača N, Luka Č, Ljubojević D, Stanaćev, V, Beuković M, Kostadinović L, Plavša N: Fatty acid composition and regression prediction of fatty acid concentration in edible chicken tissues, World's Poultry Science Journal. 2014;70:585-592, DOI: 10.1017/ S0043933914000634.

[81] Nazeer MS, Pasha TN, Shahid A, Ali Z: Effect of Yucca saponin on urease activity and development of ascites in broiler chickens. International journal of poultry science. 2002;6:174-178. DOI: http://dx.doi.org/10.3923/ijps.2002. 174.178.

[82] Patwardhan B, Gautam M: Botanical immune drugs: scope and opportunities. Drug Discovery Today. 2005;10:495.

[83] Mathe A, Essential oils: Biochemistry, production and utilization. In: T. Steiner editor. Phytogenics in Animal Nutrition.

Nottingham University Press, Nottingham. 2009;p. 71-76.

[84] Tajodini M, Samadi F, Hasani S, Hashemi RS, Samadi S: Influence of artichoke (Cynara scolymus) leaf powder on growth performance, carcass traits and blood parameters in broiler chickens. Iranian Journal of Applied Animal Science. 2015;5:141-146.

[85] Muanda F, Kone D, Dicko A, Soulimani R, Younos C: Phytochemical composition and antioxidant capacity of three malian medicinal plant parts. Evidence Based Complementary and Alternative Medicine, 2011;21-28.

[86] Caillet S, Lorenzo G, Côté J, Sylvain J, Lacroix M: Free radical-scavenging properties and antioxidant activity of fractions from cranberry products. Food and Nutrition Sciences. 2012;3:337-347. DOI:10.4236/fns.2012.33049.

[87] Ognik K, Cholewińska E, Sembratowicz I, Grela ER, Czech A: The potential of using plant antioxidants to stimulate antioxidant mechanisms in poultry. World Poultry Science Journal. 2016b;72:291-298.

[88] Dragland S, Senoo H, Wake K, Holte K, Blomhoff R: (2003) several culinary and medicinal herbs are important sources of dietary antioxidants. Nutrition Journal. 2003;33:1286-1290.

[89] Carlsen MH, Halvorsen BL, Holte K, Bøhn SK, Dragland S, Sampson L, Willey C, Senoo H, Umezono Y, Sanada C, Barikmo I, Berhe N, Willett WC, Phillips KM, Jacobs DR Jr Blomhoff R: The total antioxidant content of more than 3100 foods, beverages, spices, herbs and supplements used worldwide. Nutrition Journal. 2010;9:3.

[90] Giannenas IA, Florou-Paneri P, Botsoglou NA, Christaki E, Spais AB: Effect of supplementing feed with oregano and (or) alpha-tocopherol acetate on growth of broiler chickens and oxidative stability of meat. Journal of Animal and Feed Science. 2005;14:521-535.

[91] Florou-Paneri P, Giannenas I, Christaki E, Govaris A, Botsoglou NA: Performance of chickens and oxidative stability of the produced meat as affected by feed supplementation with oregano, vitamin C, vitamin E and their combinations. Archiv für Geflugelkunde. 2006;70:232-240.

[92] Botsoglou NA, Florou-Paneri P, Botsoglou E, Dotas V, Giannenas I, Koidis A, Mitrakos P: The effect of feeding rosemary, oregano, saffron and alpha-tocopherol acetate on hen performance and oxidative stability of eggs. South African Journal of Animal Science. 2005;35:143-151.

[93] Shirzadegan K, Falahpour P: The physicochemical properties and antioxidative potential of raw thigh meat from broilers fed a dietary medicinal herb extract mixture. Open Veterinary Journal 2014;4:69-77.

[94] Faix S, Faixová Z, Plachá I, Koppe LJ: Effect of Cinnamomum zeylanicum essential oil on antioxidative status in broiler chickens. Acta Veterinaria Hungarica. 2009;78:411-417, doi:10.1016/j.jtcme.2017.04.008.

[95] Lambert JD, Elias RJ: The antioxidant and pro-oxidant activities of green tea polyphenols: A role in cancer prevention. Archives of Biochemistry and Biophysics. 2010;501:65-72. doi:10.1016/j.abb.2010.06.013.

[96] Nyahangare ET, Hove T, Mvumi BM, Hamudikuwanda H, Belmain SR, Madzimure J, Stevenson PC: Acute mammalian toxicity of four pesticidal plants. Journal of Medicinal Plants Research. 2012; 6:2674-2680.

[97] Bernhoft, A. (Editor). Bioactive compounds in plants-benefits and risks for man and animals. The Norwegian Academy of Science and Letters, 2010.

[98] Haas J, Baungratz A, Takahashi SE, Potrich M, Lozano ER, Mazaro SM: Toxicity assessment of insecticidal plants to chicken. Revista Brasileira de Medicina do Esporte, São Paulo. 2017;19:190-196.

[99] Serrano R: Toxic plants: knowledge, medicinal uses and potential human health risks. Environment and Ecology Research. 2018;6:487-49. DOI: 10.13189/eer.2018.060509.

[100] Acamovic T, Brooker JD: Biochemistry of plant secondary metabolites and their effects in animals. Proceedings of the Nutrition Society. 2005;64:403-412.

[101] Bruneton J, Pharmacognosie. Phytochimie. Plantes médicinales, Tec et Doc, Lavoisier, Paris, France, 3rd edition, 1999.

[102] Gotardo AT, Haraguchi M, Raspantini PC, Dagli ML, Górniak SA: Toxicity of Senna occidentalis seeds in laying hens and its effects on egg production. Avian Pathology. 2017;46: 332-337, DOI:10.1080/03079457.2016.1278199.

[103] Mann K: Proteomic analysis of the chicken egg vitelline membrane. Proteomics. 2008;8:2322-2332.

[104] Nilsson JÅ, Råberg L: The resting metabolic cost of egg laying and nestling feeding in great tits. Oecologia. 2001;28:187-192.

[105] Vèzina BI, Ranaivoson A, Razafimanahaka JH, Andriafidison D, Andrianirina H, Ahamadi K, Rabearivony J, Gardner CJ: Understanding livelihoods for protected area management: Insights from northern Madagascar. Conservation and Society. 2020;18:327-339.

[106] Díaz-Zaragoza M, Carvajal-Moreno M, Méndez-Ramírez I, Chilpa-Galván NC, Ávila-González E, Flores-Ortiz CM: Aflatoxins, hydroxylated metabolites, and aflatoxicol from breast muscle of laying hens. Poultry Science. 2014;93: 3152-3162.DOI.org/10.3382/ps.2014-04240.

[107] Nelson LS, Shih RD, Balick MJ: Handbook of Poisonous and Injurious Plants. Second Edition, New York Botanical Garden Press/Springer-Verlag, New York, US, 2007.

[108] Tremaine LM, Bird JE, Quebbemann AJ: Renal tubular excretory transport of oxalate in the chicken. Journal Pharmacology and Experimental Therapy. 1985;233:7-11.

[109] Juodka R, Nainiene R, Juskiene V, Juska R, Stuoge I, Leikus R: Effects of different amounts of blue lupine *(L. Angustifolius* L.) in the diets of heavy-type turkeys on their growth rate, carcass and meat qualities. Brazilian Journal of Poultry Science. 2017;19:117-124.

[110] Benzeid H, Gouaz F, Touré AH, Bouatia M, Idrissi MOB, Draoui M: Inventory of toxic plants in Morocco: an overview of the botanical, biogeography, and phytochemistry studies. Journal of Toxicology. 2018:13. DOI.org/10.1155/2018/4563735.

[111] Mendieta MC, De Souza ADZ, Ceolin S, Vargas NRC, Ceolin T, Heck RM: Toxic plants: Importance of knowledge for realization of health education, Journal of Nursing UFPE On Line, 2014;8680-8686.

[112] Jahanian E, Jahanian R, Rahmani H, Alikhani M: Dietary supplementation of *Echinacea purpurea* powder improved performance, serum lipid profile, and yolk oxidative stability in laying hens. Journal of Applied Animal Research, 2017;45:45-51.DOI org/10.1080/09712119.2015.1091344.

Chapter 4

Use of *Bacillus Subtilis* Probiotics as Non-Antibiotic Gut Modulator and Growth Promoter in Broiler Chickens

Arbab Sikandar

Abstract

Wide range of Antibiotics is being used as feed additives in Animal industry in order to get rid from pathogens and as growth promoters in developing world. But after the suggested prohibition on using antibiotics, products such as probiotics are getting substantial importance in nutrition because of their non-resistant and non-residual possessions. Basic aim of the chapter is to highlight fruitful effects of *Bacillus Subtilis* as non-antibiotic gut modulator and growth promoter in broiler chickens. Probiotics are the living culture of microorganisms. They flourish in the gut of the host and fortify the growth of valuable commensals in the digestive tract by minimizing the destruction triggered by pathogens, boost up the immune system, supporting the integrity of the gut mucosa and maintain a stability and balance of normal microflora. Probiotics can be used as best substitute to conventional antimicrobial therapy. In addition, it has been observed that probiotics plays a role in growth enhancement by augmenting useful enzymes in the body and promote the growth of other normal commensals such as Lactobacillus and having effect on gut luminal pH. Probiotics are quite active against intestinal pathogens in several ways, viz. including improved immune elimination, competing for mucosal attachment, striving for crucial nutrients, or producing antimicrobial complexes contrary to numerous enteropathogens. It can be concluded that *B. Subtilis* has the ability to modulate gut and immune system histophysiology and histomorphology and can be used as safe antimicrobial candidate in poultry nutrition. Knowledge of such possessions of the *B. Subtilis* as probiotics and the mechanisms of action may enable the researchers to manipulate the use of such alternatives for better growth production, and safe and healthy poultry industry.

Keywords: anatomy, commercial broiler, gut, microscope, physiology, probiotics

1. Introduction

Throughout the world, domestic animals are being kept producing high-quality meat. Chicken also contributes a major portion to the animal meat source and more than 45% of the world population is potential consumers of chicken meat [1]. A gape exists between supply and demand, and some sort of discriminations are observed among the availability of protein source to the people of technological advanced countries and the underdeveloped countries. Annual meat availability per capita is 0.25 to 1.25 kg in Southern Asian Countries in comparison with 20–30 kg meat in some developed countries [2]. Current animal industry needs elevated production level and cost-effective feed conversion, which to a reliable level could be attained by the practice of precise additives. Sustained meat production can be hampered by various disease conditions especially those affecting digestive systems of the animals. Salmonellosis, colibacillosis, coccidiosis and some fungal toxins are the leading causative agents among those. Most of the diseases are transferable via food chain and have a zoonotic impact. Salmonellosisis among the foremost reasons of bacterial food poisoning in end-users (humans) in both the developing and technologically advanced countries [3]. Wide range of Antibiotics is being used in poultry sectorsin order to get rid from pathogens and as a growth promoter all over the world. The excessive use of dietary antimicrobials has caused a collective trouble, for instance the progress and growth of resistant microbes, disparity of gut commensals and drug residues in the bird's body [4]. But after the projected outlaw on practicing antibiotics in the feed, products like probiotics are getting substantial importance nutrition offered to the animals. The probiotics are well known for having non-resistant and non-residual properties [5]. Bacillus type of probiotics are being used against salmonellosis [6] and necrotic enteritis [7] and are enjoying the status of immune booster and safe growth promoter in commercial chickens.

To overcome the drawbacks of using antibiotics as feed additives, it is need of the day to find a substitute. Probiotics have the potential to be used for this purpose. Its supplementation in the feed markedly improves weight gain, carcass characteristics and amplifies the intestinal absorption area by increasing intestinal villi length and width. Microscopic modulation of mucosal morphology of the intestine is assumed to improve health indicators and production performance in broiler but the intermediate structural changes, which result into improved performance in this case, are not adequately documented. Basic aim of the chapter is to highlight fruitful effects of *Bacillus Subtilis* as non-antibiotic gut modulator and growth promoter in broiler chicken.

2. Probiotics and its properties in general

Probiotics are the living culture of microorganisms offered orally. These organisms flourish in the host gut and cause rapid activation of the intestinal functions, fortify the beneficial commensals growth in the gut by minimizing the destruction triggered by pathogens, boost up the immune system especially innate immunity, supporting the integrity of the gut mucosa and maintain a stability and balance of normal microflora and improvement of the growth performance [8, 9]. For getting determined benefit (as substitute to antibiotics and used against *Salmonella* spp), recently, de Oliveira et al. [10] recommend and advised the constant offering of probiotics (*B. subtilis*) spores or as vegetative cells. *B. Subtilis* are gram positive, chain/clumps forming rod-shaped endospore forming heterotrophic bacterium. They are facultative anaerobe and has flagella and a single chromosome that is circular in shape and positioned in cytoplasm at nucleoid region. A noticeable benefit of *B. subtilis* in feed is the permanency because it can stand with the hostile environment like low pH and intra luminal bile salt without dropping viability. *B. Subtilis* in animal nutrition is harmless probiotic. Being used extensively as a nutrition supplement in broilers due to its established immunomodulatory, enzymatic, anti-inflammatory and antioxidant activity (**Figure 1**) Bacillus can be used as best substitute to conventional antimicrobial therapy in broilers [11]. Additionally, various species of *Bacillus* organism have the ability to generate some useful

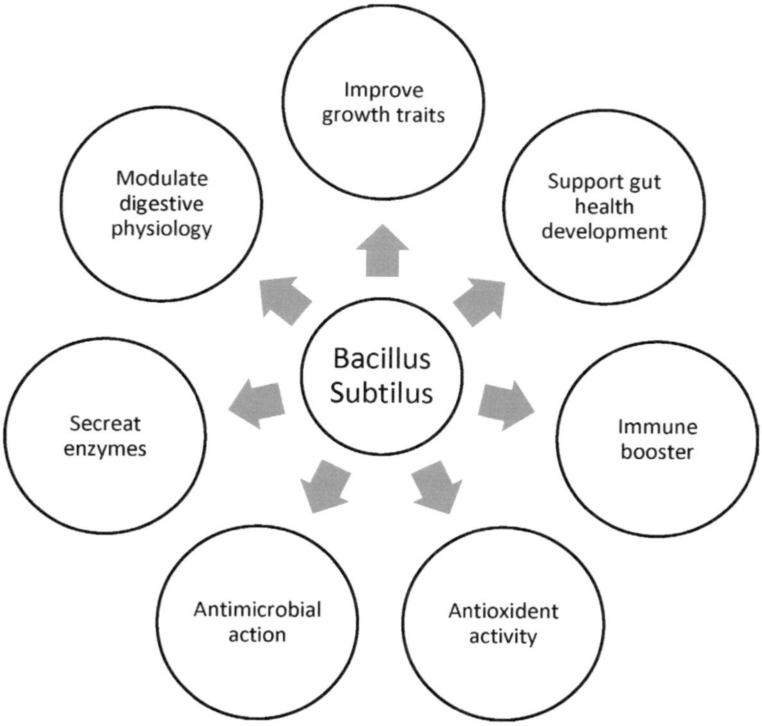

Figure 1.
Fruitful effects of B. Subtiliss *on chicken's body.*

exogenic enzymes like lipase, cellulase, protease, keratinase, xylanase and phytase [12]. These enzymes are expected to be involved in diminished gut luminal stickiness in starch less polysaccharide foods, decomposition of complex feed molecules in the host animal gut, improve nutrients absorption and decline the substrates accessible for pathogens growth. Furthermore, it is observed that *B. subtilis* plays a role in growth enhancement of other normal commensals such as *Lactobacillus* by decreasing pH of the gut luminal [13]. Probiotics are quite active against intestinal pathogens in several ways, viz. including improved immune elimination, striving for vital nutrients, opposing for attachment with mucosa, or producing antimicrobial complexes contrary to numerous pathogens in chickens [14]. The advantageous properties on improvement in digestive performance and also on immune boosting of probiotic supplements have been previously established in broilers [7].

3. Factors affecting animal performance and its possible solution

There are various exogenous and endogenous factors which weaken the performance of immune system in animals [15] and ultimately minimizing the growth production. Pathogens like bacteria, virus, parasites, fungi and harsh environmental stresses also contributing to creating adverse effects on the animal growth. To overcome these circumstances, and, to achieve maximum production, animal industry in the developing countries is using excessive amount of antibiotics as feed additives which is hazardous to human health. It is need of the day to formulate new safe ways and means in probiotics form to boost up the gut health and immune system of the animals in intensive farming systems to achieve maximum production potential and various researchers recommended the constant administration of Bacillus spores or vegetative cells (a probiotics), along with acidifiers, enzymes, prebiotics and phytobiotics as a potential substitute to antibiotics [16]. These substances are focusing the gut luminal health. As good gut health reflects better growth performance in animals.

4. Association of gut histomorphology with immunity broiler chickens

With standing a good digestive track ecosystem is a criterion for obtaining well-organized animal health, immunity, and performance. Beside nutrients digestion and absorption, the alimentary tract is playing a decisive role as barrier against everlasting attack of disease-causing microorganisms. There is a bulk of pathogenic organisms in the luminal ecosystem of the gut within ingesta. The tight junction in the lining epithelial cells not allowing any pathogens to reach the lamina propria in which a rich blood vascular system exists. In addition to the tight junction, a thick mucus layer which is secreted by the lining goblet cells also complement to maintain the immunity. Disturbance in the immune system may leads to enteritis [17]. During pathogenic bacterial infection, lymphocytes will accumulate in the lamina propria to defend the tissue against the pathogens. Other mononuclear cells including macrophages, plasma cells accompanying the lymphocytes and may cause inflammation and causing thickness in the lamina propria [18]. If the pathogen persists in the lumen then there is high possibility to deteriorate the normal physiological functions of the gut. Normal integrity of the mucosa may be deteriorated. The lining epithelium may be sloughed-off and the mucosa will become shorter and also appear denuded [19]. Thickness will be descended till remaining portions of the mucosa and even submucosa. Fluid will accumulate in the lumen and its absorption will obviously minimizes. Such stressful conditions will leads to affect the systemic immune system of the animals. Important pathogen's effect and influencing that animal effortlessly.

Salmonellosis is one of the important pathogens of chickens which may leads to potential human foodborne infection also [3, 16]. Broiler chickens assist as haulers and express seldom signs of diarrhea not like human. Both living bacteria and its endotoxins displayed similar effects on the gut mucosal surface [19]. The broiler may be perceived as showing inversely synchronizing the physiology of gut rather than showing resistance to Salmonella infection [18]. Few moderate mucosal lesions have been observed by Porter and Holt [20] after *Salmonella Enteritidis* infection in chickens as compared with those in mammals. The later species are observed to be involved in diphtheritic typhlitis, inflammation in intestine, fibrinus filled ceca, penetration of plasma cells and macrophages in the mucosa, and sloughed lining epithelial cells [21]. *S. gallinarum* may be separated from spleen and liver of the chicken [6]. Kwag et al. [21] demonstrated numerous factors through which the pathogen may add to support the gut epithelium impairment. These includes lining mucosal infiltration, production of toxin, and causing enteritis, nevertheless, the precise means for this damage is still not clear [22]. So, we hypothesize that probiotics supplementations have favorable possessions on histology of small intestine and histomorphometric parameters of different organs of broiler chickens. Reviews of this chapters will also help us to understand the influence of *B. subtilis* on selected gut and immune systems parameters of broiler chickens.

Good gut health reflects safe meat production if best management and husbandry protocol is provided to the animal. The alimentary tract is playing a decisive role in nutrient digestion and absorption also act as a defensive obstacle alongside endless violence of disease-causing microorganisms. Numerous microanatomical features determine the total surface area for absorption of the GIT. The intestinal villi and crypts microarchitecture are linked with the gut function which ultimately leads to the animal growth [23–25]. In order to assess the immune organ status under microscope in animals one needs to slaughter that animal. A prior approval from the ethical committee is utmost required to do this. Soon after humane sacrificing, the immune represented visceral organs including thymus and spleen may be grossly examined for any morphological changes and their representative samples may be collected and processed onward for histomorphometry. To identify the microstructural changes, around 2 cm segments is acquired from different segments of small and large intestines and fixed in some suitable fixatives. The same are then impregnating in paraffin to provide easy environment for micro-sectioning. The slices are afterward processed and stained with dyes namely hematoxylin and eosin along with using some other special staining materials. The prepared slides are then subjected to the process of cover slipping for everlastingly preservation [26]. Pictures obtained from the gut slides will be obtained from the suitable area under microscope fitted with digital imaging system and will be examined for determination of villus length, width, depth of crypt, surface area of villi. Villi and crypt microstructures are also required to study to determine the height of the villus: crypt depth ratio. The goblet cells numbers per villus and its variation on mucins basis viz. acidic, neutral, and mixed from and the histomorphometry (height, width and area of lymphatic tissues in one microscopic field of each section at 4X under light microscope) of immune organs (thymus and spleen) is also needs to be observed because these parameters are needed to provide some clue for immune indicator.

5. Effects of probiotics on growth performance

Probiotics are living microbes and after being supplementation to the feed, it maintains normal intestine commensal equilibrium. The probiotics has been reported to fortify the gut physiology including digestive and absorptive functions [8], which ultimately leads to obtain better growth and FCR in broilers [27, 28], turkeys [29], Pigs [30], Sheep [31], Rabbits [32], Fishes [33], Canine [34] Goats [35] and in Cattle [36]. It has been studied that developed egg weight, size and mass in layers are associated with offering Probiotics [35, 37], along with repressed cholesterol level in chickens [36, 38]. Such fruitful effects created in the organic protein source increases further its demands in the market. The end user love to approach for getting the safer organic meat from the supplier. Several findings have been revealed that direct feed microbials are possible substitutes to antibiotic growth promoters [39, 40].

6. *Bacillus Subtilis* as a probiotic in chicken industry

B. subtilis is gaining much attention towards animal nutrition in the area where animals are kept under stressful conditions such as harsh environment and food deprived locations. The stress may affect directly or indirectly the immune system of the animal body. The immune system comprising organs, tissues and cells those are responsible to maintaining integrity of the body. This system ensures the protective responses of the body to the external substance appropriately. It is observed that probiotics can defend the animals beside disease causing organisms [41] and has encouraging influence on cellular and humoral immunity [42]. Diet supplemented with *B. subtilis* showed better feed conversion ratio (FCR), statistically better mean live body weight, mean weight gains, relatively bigger breasts and reduced mortality [11, 43].

Various bacillus species produced spores that can germinate and became effective metabolically in the gastrointestinal tract, thus displaying achievement comparable to additional well-established probiotics [44]. Awad et al. [45] and Murugesan et al. [8] reported previously that probiotics strengthen the barrier task of the gut mucosa. In the past the Samanya and Yamaouchi [46] found that *B. subtilis* decreases the concentration of ammonia in blood, which ultimately results in motivation of intestinal function and reported to use *B. subtilis* in chicken's feed. In mucosa of the intestinal tract the villus height and its per field area numbers are associated to the maximum absorption capability of the gut lining cells. Enlarged gut mucosal villi is directly proportional to expand the absorptions activity of the nutrients in the GIT [24] and occurrence of small mucosal villi declines the nutrients absorption surface area which ultimately leads to lower the production performance [26]. It is recommended that in feed *B. subtilis* displayed significantly greater villus length of all the small intestinal segments in pigs [47]. Crypts are the areas where the epithelial cells of the villi originate, and deep crypt shows constant turnover of tissue and extraordinary need for fresh tissues [24, 46]. Molnar et al. [43] found that increased infiltration of lymphocytes in the gut mucosa is associated with the dietary inclusion of probiotics in broilers. Little knowledge is available in the literature to study the probiotics influence on animals [38] and there is also least information available regarding influence of various probiotics on histological alterations in gut mucosa of animals. *B. subtilis* has been reported to develop the immunity in weanling pigs [47] and the bacillus spores may cause propagation of follicular cells Peyer's patches in mice [48]. *B. subtilis* based direct feed microbial displayed the immunomodulatory effects on innate immunity in broiler chickens [49]. Molnar et al. [43] recommended the increase concentration of in fed *B. subtilis* significantly decreased the coliform bacterial population in the ileum or in the caecum of the commercial broiler chickens. *B. subtilis* displayed advantageous possessions via one or more of the following means: Reasonable exclusion and minimizing the pathogen colonization and consumption of O_2so that the anaerobic favorable bacteria may flourish [10, 50], production of useful enzymes [13], stimulation of gut physiology [45] and boosted the body immunity in broiler chickens [40].

7. Conclusion

The present work is planned to explore the importance of *Bacillus Subtilis* probiotics in broiler chicken as a feed supplementing agent. Information concerning the outcome of feed supplemented with probiotics on the growth performance, immune status and gut micro-architectural anatomy in health and disease is limited in literature. Knowledge of fruitful effects of the probiotics and the mechanisms may enable the researchers to manipulate the use of this alternatives for better growth production, and safe and healthy animal industry. Based on the latest scientific findings discussed in this chapter, the following main conclusions can be drawn that the *B. Subtilis* as probiotic:

1. Is a harmless and can be used an effective antimicrobial candidate in poultry nutrition.

2. Can withstand the harsh environment within the animal body.

3. Has the ability to modulate gut histomorphology and absorption process.

4. Fortify the enzymatic activity and digestibility of nutrients.

5. Can produce enzymes and release antioxidants.

6. Can modulate the immune system of the animal body and aid in maintenance of the body homeostasis.

7. Has better effect as growth promoter compared to antibiotic growth promoter.

Author details

Arbab Sikandar
Sub-Campus Jhang, University of Veterinary and Animal Sciences, Lahore, Pakistan

*Address all correspondence to: arbab.sikandar@uvas.edu.pk;
drarbab786@gamil.com

References

[1] Bell DD, Weaver Jr. WD. Commercial Chicken meat and egg production, 5th edi. Springer Science plus Business media, New Delhi, India, 2007.

[2] Singh RA. Poultry Production. 3rd edi. Kalyani Publishers, New Delhi-India, 2006.

[3] Adley CC, Ryan MP. The nature and extent of foodborne disease. In Antimicrobial food packaging 2016 Jan 1 (pp. 1-10). Academic Press.

[4] Diarra MS, Malouin F. 2104. Antibiotics in Canadian poultry productions and anticipated alternatives. Frontiers in Micro. doi: 10.3389/fmicb.2014.00282.

[5] Kocher A, 2005. AGP alternatives-part IV. Poultry production without AGPs- Challenges and solutions. Worl Poult. 21 (9): 32-33.

[6] Sikandar A, Zaneb H, Nasir A, Adil M, Ali HM, Muhammad M, Rehman T, Rehman A, Rehman HF. Effects of *Bacillus Subtilis* on performance, immune system and gut in Salmonella-challenged broilers. South African Journal of Animal Science. 2020;50(5):654-662.

[7] TactacanGB, Schmidt JK, Miille MJ, Jimenez DR. 2013. A *Bacillus Subtilis* (QST 713) spore-based probiotic for necrotic enteritis control in broiler chickens. The J of Applied Poult Resr. 22 (4): 825-831.

[8] Murugesan GR., Gabler NK, Persia ME. 2014. Effects of direct-fed microbial supplementation on broiler performance, intestinal nutrient transport and integrity under experimental conditions with increased microbial challenge. Brit Poul Sci. 55 : (1) 89-97.

[9] Park JH, Kim IH. 2014a. Supplemental effect of probiotic *Bacillus Subtilis* B2A on productivity, organ weight, intestinal Salmonella microflora, and breast meat quality of growing broiler chicks. Poult Sci. 93:2054-2059

[10] de Oliveira JE, van der Hoeven-Hangoor 1E. van de Linde IB, Montijn RC, van der Vossen JMBM. 2014. In ovo inoculation of chicken embryos with probiotic bacteria and its effect on posthatch Salmonella susceptibility . Poult Sci. 93 :818-829.

[11] Dersjant-Li Yueming, Awati A, Kromm C, Evans C. 2014. A direct fed microbial containing a combination of three-strain Bacillus spp. can be used as an alternative to feed antibiotic growth promoters in broiler production. J. of Appli. Ani Nutr. 2; 01-06.

[12] Shah KR, Bhatt SA. 2011. Purification and characterization of lipase from *Bacillus Subtilis* Pa2. J Biochem Tech. 3:292-295.

[13] Hosoi T, Ametani A, Kiuchi K, Kaminogawa S. 2000. Improved growth and viability of lactobacilli in the presence of *Bacillus Subtilis* (natto), catalase, or subtilisin. Can J Microbiol. 46:892-897.

[14] Cartman ST, La Ragione RM, Woodward MJ. 2008. *Bacillus Subtilis* spores germinate in the chicken gastrointestinal tract. Appl Environ Microbiol. 74:5254-5258.

[15] Esser C, editor. Environmental influences on the immune system. Vienna, Austria:: Springer; 2016 Feb 4.

[16] Tellez G, Pixley C, Wolfenden R, Layton S, Hargis B. 2012. Probiotics/ direct fed microbials for Salmonella control in poultry. Food Res Int. 45:628-633.

[17] Liu W, Ruan T, Ji X, Ran D, Sun J, Shi H, Prinz RA, Sun J, Pan Z, Jiao X,

Xu X. The Gli1-Snail axis contributes to Salmonella Typhimurium-induced disruption of intercellular junctions of intestinal epithelial cells. Cellular microbiology. 2020 Aug;22(8):e13211.

[18] Tellez G, Kogut MH, Hargis BM. 1994. Eimeria tenella or Eimeria adenoeides: induction of morphological changes and increased resistance to Salmonella enteritidis infection in Leghorn chicks. Poult Sci. 73:396-401.

[19] Sikandar A, Cheema AH, Younus M, Aslam A, Zaman MA, Rehman T. Histopathological and serological studies on paratuberculosis in catle and bufaloes. Pakistan Veterinary Journal. 2012;4:547-551

[20] Porter Jr, RE and Holt PS. Effect of induced molting on the severity of intestinal lesions caused by Salmonella enteritidis infections in chickens. Avian Diseases. 1993; 37: 1009-1016.

[21] Kwag SI, Bae DH, Cho JK, Lee HS, Ku BG, Kim BH, Cho GJ, Lee YJ. 2008. Characteristics of persistent Salmonella Enteritidis strains in two integrated broiler chicken operations of Korea. J. Vet. Med. Sci. 70:1031-1035.

[22] Mehta, A., S. Singh, V. Dhawan, and N. K. Ganguly. 1998. Intestinal mucosal lipid peroxidation and absorptive function in Salmonella typhimurium mediated intestinal infection. Mol. Cell. Biochem. 178:345-352.

[23] Sikandar A, Zaneb H, Younus M, Masood S, Aslam A, Khattak F, et al. Effect of sodium butyrate on performance, immune status, microarchitecture of small intestinal mucosa and lymphoid organs in broiler chickens. Asian-Australasian Journal of Animal Sciences. 2017c;30(5):690

[24] Awad WA, Molnar A, Aschenbach JR, Ghareeb K, Khayal B, Hess C , Liebhart D, Dublecz K, Hess M. 2014. Campylobacter infection in chickens modulates the intestinal epithelial barrier function. Innate Immunity DOI: 10.1177/175342 5914521648.

[25] Iqbal S, Hafeez A, Sikandar A, Khan I, Ashraf S, Khan RU, Tufarelli V, Laudadio V. Feeding of Phytobiotics and Exogenous Protease in Broilers: Comparative Effect on Nutrient Digestibility, Bone Strength and Gut Morphology. Agriculture 2021; 11: 228.

[26] Sikandar 2018. Histopathology: An Old Yet Important Technique in Modern Science http://dx.doi.org/10.5772/intechopen.76908

[27] Wu LY, Tan RB, Shi KJ. 2008. Effect of a dried *Bacillus Subtilis* culture on gosling growth performance. Bri Poult Sci. 49, 4: 418- 422.

[28] El Jeni R, Dittoe DK, Olson EG, Lourenco J, Corcionivoschi N, Ricke SC, Callaway TR. Probiotics and Potential Applications for Alternative Poultry Production Systems. Poultry Science. 2021 Mar 26:101156.

[29] Nair DV, Thomas JV, Dewi G, Brannon J, Noll SL, Johnson TJ, Cox RB, Johny AK. Propionibacterium freudenreichiifreudenreichii B3523 reduces cecal colonization and internal organ dissemination of multidrug-resistant Salmonella Heidelberg in Finishing Turkeys. Journal of Applied Poultry Research. 2021 Mar 1;30(1):100107.

[30] Kwak, M.J., Tan, P.L., Oh, J.K., Chae, K.S., Kim, J., Kim, S.H., Eun, J.S., Chee, S.W., Kang, D.K., Kim, S.H. and Whang, K.Y., 2021. The effects of multispecies probiotic formulations on growth performance, hepatic metabolism, intestinal integrity and fecal microbiota in growing-finishing pigs. Animal Feed Science and Technology, 274, p.114833.

[31] Devyatkin, Vladimir, Alexey Mishurov, and Evgenia Kolodina.

"Probiotic effect of *Bacillus Subtilis* B-2998D, B-3057D, and Bacillus licheniformis B-2999D complex on sheep and lambs." Journal of Advanced Veterinary & Animal Research 8, no. 1 (2021).

[32] Helal F, El-Badawi A, El-Naggar S, Shourrap M, Aboelazab O, Hafsa SA. Probiotics role of Saccharomyces cerevisiae and *Bacillus Subtilis* in improving the health status of rabbits' gastrointestinal tract. Bulletin of the National Research Centre. 2021 Dec;45(1):1-9.

[33] Milián-Sorribes MC, Martínez-Llorens S, Cruz-Castellón C, Jover-Cerdá M, Tomás-Vidal A. Effect of fish oil replacement and probiotic addition on growth, body composition and histological parameters of yellowtail (Seriola dumerili). Aquaculture Nutrition. 2021 Feb;27(1):3-16.

[34] Gómez-Gallego C, Forsgren M, Selma-Royo M, Nermes M, Collado MC, Salminen S, Beasley S, Isolauri E. The Composition and Diversity of the Gut Microbiota in Children Is Modifiable by the Household Dogs: Impact of a Canine-Specific Probiotic. Microorganisms. 2021 Mar;9(3):557.

[35] Maake TW, Adeleke M, Aiyegoro OA. Effect of lactic acid bacteria administered as feed supplement on the weight gain and ruminal pH in two South African goat breeds. Transactions of the Royal Society of South Africa. 2021 Jan 28:1-6.

[36] Mombach MA, da Silva Cabral L, Lima LR, Ferreira DC, e Pedreira BC, Pereira DH. Association of ionophores, yeast, and bacterial probiotics alters the abundance of ruminal microbial species of pasture intensively finished beef cattle. Tropical Animal Health and Production. 2021 Dec;53(1):1-1.

[37] Abdelqader A, Al-Fataftah A, Das G. 2013. Effects of dietary *Bacillus Subtilis* and inulin supplementation on performance, eggshell quality, intestinalmorphology and microflora composition of laying hens in the late phase of production. Anim Feed Sci Technol. 179: 103-111.

[38] Santoso U, Tanaka K, Ohtani S, Sakaida M, 2001. Effect of fermented product from *Bacillus Subtilis* on feed conversion efficiency, lipid accumulation and ammonia production in broiler chicks. Asian–Aust J Anim Sci. 14: 333-333.

[39] Amerah AM, Jansen van RC, Plumstead PW, Kromm C, Dunham S. 2013a. Effect of feeding diets containing a probiotic or antibiotic on broiler performance, intestinal mucosa-associated avian pathogenic E. coli and litter water-soluble phosphorus. Journal of Applied Animal Nutrition, Vol. 1,7;1 of 7. doi:10.1017/jan.2013.4.

[40] Sikandar A, Zaneb H, Younus M, Masood S, Aslam A, Shah M, et al. Growth performance, immune status and organ morphometry in broilers fed *Bacillus Subtilis*-supplemented diet. South African Journal of Animal Science. 2017a;47(3):378-388

[41] Lee M. 2002. Microbial dynamics of the broiler intestinal tract, The Elanco Global Enteritis Symposium, July 9-11.

[42] Koenen ME, Kramer J, Van Der Hulst R, Heres L, Jeurissen SHM, Boersma WJA. 2004. Immunomodulation by probiotic lactobacilli in layer- and meat-type chickens. Brit Poult Sci. 45: 355-366.

[43] Molnar RAK, Podmaniczky B, Kurti P, Tenk I, Glavits R, Virag Gy. Szabo ZS. 2011. Effect of different concentrations of *Bacillus Subtilis* on growth performance, carcase quality, gut microflora and immune response of broiler chickens. Brit Poult Sci. 52: 658—665.

[44] Tam NKM, Uyen NQ, Hong HA, Duc LH, Hoa TT, Serra CR, Henriques AO, Cutting SM. 2006. The intestinal life cycle of *Bacillus Subtilis* and close relatives. J Bacteriol. 188:2692-2700.

[45] Awad WA, Ghreeb K, Nitsch S, Pasteiner S, Abdel-Raheem S, Bohm J. 2008. Effects of dietary inclusion of prebiotic, probiotic and symbiotic on the intestinal glucose absorption of broiler chickens. Int J Poult Sci. 7: 686-691.

[46] SamanyaM, Yamauchi K. 2002. Histological alterations of intestinal villi in chickens fed dried *Bacillus Subtilis* var. natto. Comparat Bioche and Physio, Part A, 133: 95-104.

[47] Lee H, Ingalea SL, Kima JS, Kima KH, Lokhandea A, Kimb EK, Kwona IK, Kimc YH, Chae BJ. 2014. Effects of dietary supplementation with *Bacillus Subtilis* LS1-2 fermentation biomass on growth performance, nutrientdigestibility, cecal microbiota and intestinal morphology of weanling pigs. Ani Feed Sci and Tech. 188:102– 110.

[48] Huang JM, LA Ragione, RM, Nunez A. Cutting SM. 2008. Immunostimulatory activity of Bacillus spores. FEMS Immunology and Medical Microbiology, 5: 195-203.

[49] Lee K-W, Li G, Lillehoj HS, Lee S-H, Jang SI, Babu US, Lillehoj EP, Neumann AP, Siragusa GR.2011.*Bacillus Subtilis*-based direct-fed microbials augment macrophage function in broiler chickens. Res.Vet. Sci. 91: 87-91

[50] Knap I, Kehlet AB, Bennedsen M, Mathis GF, Hofacre CL, Lumpkins BS, Jensen MM, Raun M, Lay A. 2011. *Bacillus Subtilis* (DSM17299) significantly reduces Salmonella in broilers. Poult Sci. 90 :1690-1694.

Chapter 5

Perspective Chapter: Using Feed Additives to Eliminate Harmful Effects of Heat Stress in Broiler Nutrition

László Babinszky, Csaba Szabó and Márta Horváth

Abstract

Global warming is one of the major challenges for mankind, with animal breeding one of the most affected sectors in the agricultural industry. High ambient temperatures negatively affect all domestic animals. While it is true that pork and dairy production suffer the consequences of heat waves, it is actually the poultry industry which is hit the hardest by the heat stress poultry must endure due to hotter weather. Consequently, we have a fundamental interest in reducing and/or eliminating the negative effects of climate change, i.e. prolonged high ambient temperatures. The aim of this chapter is to present the adverse effects of heat stress on energy metabolism, anti- and pro-oxidant capacity and production in birds. A further goal is to show how various feed additives (e.g. vitamin A, C and E, selenium, zinc, betaine, plant extract, and probiotics) can reduce the negative effects of heat stress. Based on the large number of recent scientific findings, the following conclusions were drawn: Using fat in the diet (up to 5%) can reduce heat production in livestock. Vitamins (e.g. A, E and C) are capable of reacting with free radicals. Vitamin E and Vitamin C, Zn, and Se supplementation improved antioxidant parameters. Antioxidant potential of vitamins and micro minerals is more efficient in combination under heat stress in poultry nutrition. Plant extracts (e.g. oregano) could decrease the negative effects of heat stress on antioxidant enzyme activity due to its antioxidant constituents. Betaine reduces heat production in animals at high ambient temperatures. While acute heat stress induces a drop in feed intake, with the resulting increased nutrient demand leading to weight loss, if heat stress is prolonged, adaptation will occur. Probiotics and vitamins (C and E) seem to be the most effective means to reduce the negative effects of heat stress.

Keywords: Broiler, Feed additives, Heat stress, Antioxidant status, Performance

1. Introduction

Global warming is one of the major challenges for mankind, with animal breeding one of the most affected sectors in the agricultural industry. The impacts of increasing environmental temperatures on livestock will most likely differ from place to place, depending on latitude, geographical features and local farming systems [1–3].

High ambient temperatures negatively affect all domestic animals, but in addition to pork and dairy production, perhaps the poultry industry is hit the hardest. In 2020, the world's broiler meat production amounted to about 100.81 million metric tons, and is forecasted to increase to about 101.02 million metric tons by 2021 [4]. According to FAO data [5], total egg production in the world was 1.528 billion units in 2018. In 2019, this figure reached 1.577 billion.

These statistics clearly show that broiler meat and egg production play a crucial role in the global supply of animal origin foodstuffs.

Thus, we have a fundamental interest in reducing and/or eliminating the negative effects of climate change, i.e. prolonged high ambient temperature. The main question is, what tools do we have to reduce the harmful effects of high environmental temperatures-especially in the case of heat stress? A solution for prevention of heat stress in animals includes biological (e.g. genetics, thermal conditioning, nutrition) [6, 7] or keeping technology devices (e.g. air conditioning, intensive ventilation, humidification) [8]. However, housing methods are expensive and the service costs are high. Therefore, reducing the biochemical and physiological negative effects of heat stress with different nutritional tools is one of the primary interests for the economical production of food produced from animals.

According to Babinszky et al. [9], basically the following nutritional possibilities are available to eliminate the harmful effects of the heat stress:

- reduce animal's own heat production (e.g. feeding more dietary fat);
- compensate for the lower nutrient supply; (e.g. feeding more concentrated diets); and
- mitigate heat stress induced metabolic changes (e.g. using different feed additives: vitamins, micro minerals).

It should, however, be noted that during severe heat stress, these methods should be used in combination in order to maintain the production performance of the farm animals and the quality of their products [9]. While this chapter focuses on the third option, i.e. the use of feed additives, we would like to emphasize that whatever feeding method we use, we need to be aware of the changes in the intermediate metabolism of farm animals caused by heat stress, because without this knowledge, there is no effective defense against high ambient temperatures.

Therefore, the aim of this chapter is to summarize the adverse effects of heat stress on energy metabolism, anti- and pro-oxidant capacity, and production in birds. A further goal is to show how various feed additives (vitamin A, C and E, selenium, zinc, betaine, plant extract, and probiotics) can reduce the negative effects of heat stress.

2. Methodology of the literature review

The methodology of the literature review was basically the same as the internationally applied methodology used in animal science. Firstly relevant literature was searched. This follows by evaluation of sources. The third step was identifying the database and gaps in the published scientific findings, than setup the outline structure. Finally the literature review was written.

The literature searching was based on the keywords, using university database, own department data collection on the research field of heat stress, and different international scientific databases of life sciences, animal science and Google Scholar.

In each of the studied paper or book chapter, we asked the same questions as, for example:

What was the aim and methodology of the particular publication (in this case: what kind of heat stress was applied, how many animals were included in the experiment per treatment, whether there were repetitions, what dietary treatments (type of feed additives and their concentration in the diet) were used, what parameters were measured, what was the statistical analysis applied, etc.), furthermore, whether experimental data were correctly evaluated, what results were presented by the authors and what main conclusions were drawn from the data.

To have more clear information on effectiveness of various feed supplements in case of production parameters: daily gain (g/d), average daily gain (g/d) and feed conversion ratio (kg diet/kg gain), the so called mitigation capacity was calculated using the following formula:

Mitigation capacity of a certain trait (%) = (measured value in HS environment and fed with the experimental diet – measured value in HS environment and fed with the control diet)/(measured value in TN environment and fed with the control diet–measured value in HS environment and fed with the control diet) x 100 (1)

where: HS = heat stress; TN = thermoneutral.

All collected information (data) was placed in a large work database. This information formed the basis of the subchapter titles of our review chapter and of the chapter outline. Based on this information, the evaluation of research data from more than 90 publications started. The writing of the review chapter then began, including the drawing of main conclusions as well. The investigated and systematized research findings are summarized in tables.

3. Heat production of animals and heat stress

It is well known that heat production of animals is the sum total of non-productive energy utilized by the animal and of the energy lost in the course of transformation dietary nutrients [10]. Animals use this so called non-productive energy for maintenance (i.e. satisfy the energy requirement for the maintenance of body temperature, the functioning of the nervous system, the organs, for minimal activity, etc.) [10]. The extra heat produced in the course of digestion, excretion and metabolism of nutrients is called the heat increment. It is also well known that within a certain range of ambient temperature - with unvarying feed and nutrient intake - the total heat production of the animal remains constant. This temperature range is called the thermoneutral zone. The general scheme of the relationship between ambient temperature and heat production of livestock can be seen in **Figure 1** [10].

In a thermoneutral environment, the heat production of the animal is at the minimum, and thus the dietary energy can be used for production (growth, egg and milk production) efficiently [9, 10]. Therefore, whenever the daily amount of energy intake changes, the temperature range of the thermoneutral zone is changed, too. So, if for some reason the animal leaves the thermoneutral zone, this result in an increased heat production by the animal. This means that there is more loss of energy, and in consequence, less energy remains for production and moreover the efficiency of energy utilization deteriorates too. The upper and lower critical temperatures for poultry are summarized in **Table 1** [11].

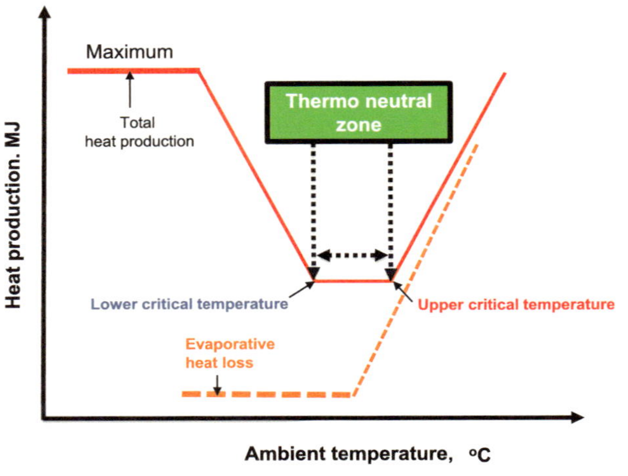

Figure 1.
Relationship between ambient temperature and heat production of livestock [10].

	Lower	Upper
	Critical temperatures (°C)	
1-day-old chicken	32	35
Finishing broiler	16	26
1-day-old turkey	35	38
Finishing turkey	16	26
Laying hen	16	27–29

Table 1.
Recommended thermal conditions for poultry [11].

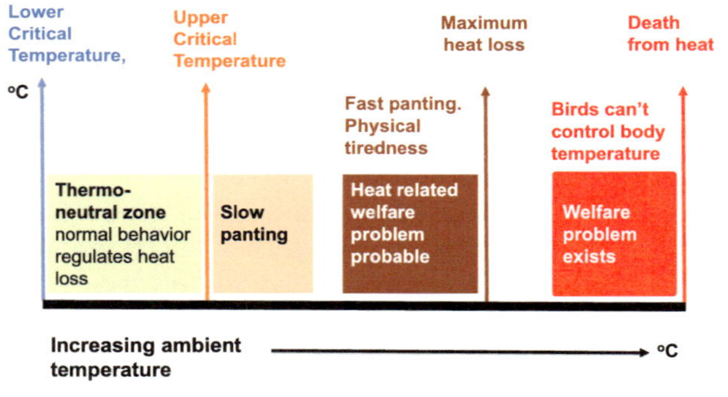

Figure 2.
The effect of increasing ambient temperature on birds [12].

The general scheme of the relationship between broiler behavior and the increasing ambient temperature is shown in **Figure 2** [12].

As can be seen in **Figure 2**, in the thermoneutral zone, birds can lose heat at a controlled rate using normal behavior [12]. Between the lower and upper temperatures, there is no heat stress and body temperature remains constant. If the environmental temperature exceeds the upper critical temperature, birds must lose heat actively by panting. However, it should be noted that panting is a normal response to heat and is not initially considered a welfare problem [12]. However, as temperatures increase, the rate of panting increases. If heat production is greater than maximum heat loss, birds may die due to heat stress. In other words, heat stress occurs when the body cannot get rid of excess heat.

It is well established that heat stress increases the energy cost of maintenance and adversely affects productive and reproductive performance. In a hot environment, the respiration rate in birds can increase 10–20 times, causing increased CO_2 loss through the lungs [13]. This loss results in an increase in blood pH and this can upset the acid–base balance, which can impair the health and performance of birds [14–16].

There are usually two types of heat stress, acute and chronic heat stress. Acute heat stress refers to a short and rapid increase in environmental temperature (a few hours), whereas under chronic heat stress, high temperatures persist for more extended periods (several days) [17].

Heat stress exposed animals can use different ways to maintain thermoregulation and homeostasis. They can increase radiant, convective and evaporative heat loss by vasodilatation and perspiration [18]. However, birds have an extra mechanism which is promote heat exchange between their bodies and the environment. These are the air sacs. Air sacs are very useful especially during panting, as they promote air circulation on surfaces and consequently, the evaporative loss of heat [19, 20].

Unfortunately, there are only few scientific papers that report on the heat production and the heat loss of heat-exposed birds. Consequently, there is only a limited number of scientific publications that report on nutritional possibilities for reducing the heat production of birds under heat stress.

Syafwan et al. [21] concluded in their excellent review that the heat production of broilers is particularly high due to the high growth rate and the high daily feed intake. Developments in the genetic selection of meat-type birds has led to rapid growth and a high metabolic rate, which is accompanied by a higher heat production level due to increased feed intake [22]. Therefore, it can be stated that high genetic capacity hybrid broilers (so called "improved chicken") are much more sensitive to a hot environment than their unimproved counterparts.

Summarizing the relevant scientific findings, it can be stated that in practical animal agriculture, and especially in factory farming, it is particularly difficult to keep animals in a thermoneutral zone. Therefore, in order to reduce the negative effect of heat stress, it is important to use nutritional tools in addition to technical devices.

4. Reduction of heat production by nutritional tools

4.1 Using fat in the diets

It is well known that if more fat is used in pig diets in high ambient temperature, the total heat production of the animals reduces significantly. Babinszky et al. [23] concluded from their study that lactating sows fed a high level of dietary fat (125 g fat/kg diet) produce significantly less heat than those fed a carbohydrate rich (low-fat level) diet. Babinszky [10] is also concluded, that the energetic efficiency of milk production was improved, when sows received high dietary fat diet (125 g/kg diet). This phenomenon can be explained by the fact that synthesizing milk fat from dietary fat is more efficient than it's synthesizing from dietary carbohydrates.

In poultry nutrition, relative limited literature data are available on fat feeding against heat stress and its effect on heat production of birds. Das et al. [24], in an excellent review, stated that heat stress may be combated by adding fat and reducing crude protein in poultry diets. Higher energy diets were effective in partially mitigating the effects of heat stress in poultry. This can be explained by the fact that during metabolism, fat produces a lower heat increment than protein and carbohydrates [25].

In other studies, it was concluded that supplementation of fat in the poultry diet increase the nutrient utilization in the gastrointestinal tract by lowering the rate of food passage [26] and also helps increase the energy value of the other feed constituents [27, 28]. Feeding a high fat diet (up to 5%) to heat-exposed broilers reduces heat production. This result occurs because the heat increment of fat is lower than that of either proteins or carbohydrates [21, 25, 29, 30].

4.2 Using vitamin C in chicken diet to change energy metabolism

Because the animal body derives all its energy from oxidation, the magnitude of energy metabolism can be determined from the amount of carbon-dioxide produced and oxygen consumed. The ratio of the volumes of carbon dioxide produced to oxygen consumed is called the respiratory quotient (RQ) [31]. The respiratory quotients are: for protein: 0.809; for fat: 0.711; for starch: 1.000; for sugar: 1.000; and for glucose: 1.000, respectively [32]. If the RQ value is equal to 1.00, this means that e.g. burning 1 g of starch produces as much carbon dioxide as oxygen is needed to burn it (0.829 liter CO_2/0.829 liter O_2).

However, it should also be noted that RQ values significantly higher than 1 can be achieved if the animals convert the carbohydrate to fat, since in this case oxygen-poor fat is formed from oxygen-rich glucose. During starvation, the RQ value is less than 0.7 [31].

As it can be seen above, the RQ may provide valuable information about the metabolic processes in the body. Therefore, RQ values are very often determined in respiratory studies.

McKee et al. [33] investigated the effect of vitamin C on different variables of energy metabolism of young heat exposed chickens in indirect calorimeters. The experiment started at day 9 and lasted until day 17 posthatch. In this study, CO_2 production and O_2 consumption were measured in the thermoneutral zone (27.7°C) and in a hot environment (34°C). On the basis of these values, RQ and heat production were calculated daily through day 17 of the experiment. The basal diet was supplemented by a 150 mg/kg diet of ascorbic acid (vitamin C). They found that heat exposure lowered ($P < 0.001$) the respiratory quotient. Heat-exposed birds consuming the ascorbic acid supplemented diet expressed lower respiratory quotients than their unsupplemented counterparts. The authors concluded that this effect resulted from a nonsignificant increase in O_2 consumption and decrease in CO_2 production. They also concluded that further investigations are needed to determine whether the ascorbic acid-induced change in the RQ value towards 0.70 reflects an increase in protein or lipid catabolism or both. In further study, the effect of ascorbic acid on the energy metabolism and heat production of domestic animals should also be elucidated.

Despite the many open questions, based on the findings made by McKee et al. in their study, it seems that supplemental ascorbic acid may influence the body energy stores during periods of reduced energy intake (during heat stress).

4.3 Using betaine as feed additive in the diet

Betaine chemical structure ($C_5H_{11}NO_2$) contains three methyl groups which play a role in transmethylation reactions [34]. Betaine (trimethylglycine) is an intermediate metabolite in the catabolism of choline which can modify osmolarity, act as a methyl donor, and has potential lipotropic effects [9]. As a by-product of sugar beet processing, betaine is commercially available as a feed additive [35]. Currently, betaine is available in several purified forms (anhydrous, monophosphate and hydrochloride betaine) [36].

Betaine mainly functions as an osmolyte and a methyl-group donor [37]. Under heat stress, betaine plays an important role in cellular osmotic regulation, preventing dehydration by increasing the water-holding capacity of cells. It helps in maintaining the protective osmolytic activity in birds under heat stress. Betaine may promote various intestinal microbes against osmotic variations and this results in improve microbial fermentation activity [38]. Furthermore, betaine is also found to have anti-inflammatory properties and improves intestinal function [39].

Because betaine influences fat and protein deposition, it can also be used to improve carcass quality and reduce fatty livers. Schrama et al. [40] showed that energy retention in pigs improves over time following the supplementation of betaine to the diet. They also found that under thermoneutral conditions, dietary betaine supplementation (1.23g/kg diet) reduced the total heat production of pigs. They suggest the same concentration of betaine in poultry diet, as well.

These scientific findings suggest that betaine may be suitable for reducing heat production in livestock (e.g. in poultry) at high ambient temperatures. However, only few research results have been published in this area to date. Therefore, further studies are needed to determine the impact of betaine on heat production in animals under high ambient temperature.

Another problem is that many of published papers are not clear on the source of betaine used (natural, extracted betaine anhydrous or synthetic betaine hydrochloride). The source is important, as it is likely that the efficacies of the different betaine sources differ.

5. Effects of heat stress on anti- and prooxidant status in birds. Mitigation using different feed additives

5.1 Anti- and prooxidant status

5.1.1 Impacts of heat stress

Increased environmental temperature caused increased lipid peroxidation (as well as induced formation of malondialdehyde (MDA), which is an indicator for lipid peroxidation). Therefore, the antioxidant defense system is altered [41–43].

According to the latest research, the elimination of the free radicals activates three level antioxidant systems (**Figure 3**, based on Babinszky et al. [10]).

Elimination is done by the first level of the antioxidant system which functions at the same time as the detoxification and regeneration pathways of the second level. The third level starts working after damage has been done, to repair and eliminate damaged cells. This first level (direct enzymatic pathway) includes the neutralization of the oxygen and nitrogen centred free radicals by enzymes. The second level includes the detoxification and regeneration reactions of the small molecule antioxidants. The third level is activated when damaged systems (proteins, DNA) have to be repaired and/or removed from the cells by chaperones and DNA-repair enzymes.

In general, it can be concluded that a large amount of Reactive Oxygen Species (ROS) causes disruption of mitochondrial function, increased lipid peroxidation,

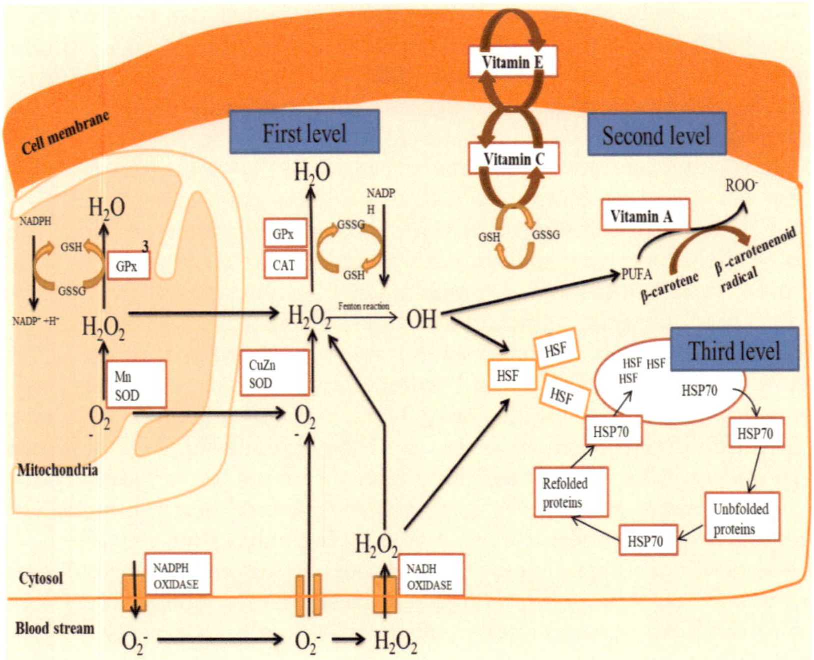

Figure 3.
Three level antioxidant system. Based on Babinszky et al. [10]. CAT = catalase; Cu SOD = copper superoxide dismutase; GPx = glutathione peroxidase; GR=glutathione reductase; GSH = glutathione; GSSG = glutathione disulphide; H_2O = water; H_2O_2 = hydrogen peroxide; HSF = heat shock factors; HSP70 = heat shock protein 70; Mn SOD = manganese superoxide dismutase; NADH=nicotinamide-adenine-dinucleotide; $NADP^+$ = oxidised nicotinamide-adenine-dinucleotide-phosphate, NADPH=nicotinamide-adenine-dinucleotide-phosphate, O_2^- = superoxide anion radical; OH = hydroxyl radical; PUFA = polyunsaturated fatty acids; ROO^- = peroxyl radical.

and decreased the concentration of so called antioxidant vitamins, furthermore induce stress gene expression, and finally it leads to dysfunction in antioxidant enzymes and also causes DNA damage.

According to Yang et al. [44] in heat stressed broilers (35°C for 3h/day), the activity of the mitochondrial respiratory chain is reduced, which led to over-production of ROS. This situation results in lipid peroxidation and oxidative stress in the birds.

In another study [7] lipid peroxidation and superoxide dismutase (SOD) activity was measured in broilers under heat stress (32°C for 6 h/day). The results showed that high temperature disturbed the equilibrium between the synthesis and catabolism of ROS production. Glutathione peroxidase (GPx) and SOD activity increased and catalyze (CAT) activity decreased under heat stress (34°C 5 h/day from d28 to d38) [45].

ROS production reduced Vitamin A and E levels. Vitamin C concentration decreased under heat stress in poultry [46]. It has been reported that heat stress increased zinc (Zn) mobilization from tissues, and thus may cause marginal Zn deficiency and increase requirements [47]. According to Zeng et al. [48, 49], SOD, MDA, CAT activity and the total antioxidant capacity (T-AOC) in Muscovy duck liver increased under short term heat stress (39°C for 1 hour then 3-hour recovery at20°C). The same results were found in broilers [50]. During heat stress in broilers, the serum concentrations of Vitamin C, E, A, iron (Fe), and Zn decreased, while the copper (Cu) concentration increased [51].

5.1.2 Using feed additives

5.1.2.1 Vitamin supplementation

High environmental temperature decreases the concentrations of vitamins and micro minerals in serum and increases excretion [52]; therefore, supplementation of direct or indirect antioxidant compounds (e.g. vitamins and micro nutrients) at higher levels is commonly recommended. These additives support mechanisms against lipid peroxidation, improve immune status and performance.

5.1.2.1.1 Vitamin E

Vitamin E functions as a fat-soluble antioxidant which protects cellular and membrane lipids from peroxidation-catalyzed free radicals due to heat stress. In cell membranes and lipoproteins, the essential antioxidant function of Vitamin E is to trap ROO^- and to break the chain reaction of lipid peroxidation. While it cannot prevent their formation, it can reduce the formation of secondary radicals [53]. Vitamin E is known as the first line of defense against lipid peroxidation caused by heat stress. It has free radical quenching activity and attacks free radicals in an early stage. When feed was supplemented with Vitamin E (200-250 mg/kg feed), the serum concentration of Vitamins E and A increased in serum and MDA concentration decreased under long term heat stress [51]. Maini et al. [54] reported that CAT, GR, GSH, MDA and SOD level decreased under heat stress due to Vitamin E supplementation. Short term heat stress increased the concentration of Zn in serum when the diet was supplemented with Vitamin E [55] (**Table 2**, [56]).

Author(s)	Spices	Duration of the study	Environmental temperature	Amount of vitamin supplementation	Effects on antioxidant status
Kucuk et al. [57]	broiler	1–42 day	34°C (24 h/day)	Vitamin A: 15 000 IU/kg diet	↓MDA
Mahmoud and Edens, [58]	broiler	1–42 day	30 °C (3.5 h/ for 3 days)	Vitamin C: 500 mg/kg diet	↑plasma ascorbic acid concentration ↓Hsp70 expression
Sahin et al. [51]	Japanese quail	10–40day	34°C (24 h/day)	Vitamin E: 250 mg/kg diet	↑Vitamin E, A concentration in serum ↓ MDA
Maini et al. [54]	broiler	1–49 day	38.6 ± 1.3 °C (24 h/day)	Vitamin E: 200 mg/kg diet	↓CAT, GR, GSH, MDA, SOD
Harsini et al. [55]	broiler	1–49 day	37°C (8 h/day)	Vitamin E: 250 mg/kg diet	↑Zn concentration in serum

CAT = catalase concentration in blood; GR = glutathione reductase concentration in blood; GSH = reduced glutathione concentration in blood; MDA = malondialdehyde concentration in blood; SOD = superoxide dismutase concentration in blood; Zn = zinc.
↑ Increase; ↓ decrease.

Table 2.
Effects of selected vitamin supplementation under heat stress based on different studies [56].

5.1.2.1.2 Vitamin C

Vitamin C protects against oxidative stress-induced cellular damage in the presence of scavenging ROS, and is capable itself of inhibiting lipid peroxidation in plasma. Ascorbic acid can directly scavenge radicals in the aqueous compartment. Ascorbate can scavenge O_2^-, H_2O_2, the OH, hypochlorous acid, aqueous ROO^-, and singlet oxygen. Under its antioxidant activity, ascorbate has a two-electron reduction [53]. Although chickens are known to synthesize ascorbic acid in the kidney, increased supplementation has proved beneficial effects in broilers reared under heat stress [59]. Ascorbic acid is actively absorbed. This active transport is supported by the sodium electrochemical gradient. However, the vitamin C requirements increase under heat stress. According to different studies, ascorbic acid supplementation (200 mg/kg feed) caused a significant increase in plasma ascorbic acid levels [59, 60] in broilers under heat stress. This indicates that the higher Vitamin C concentrations in the broiler diet could be used against heat stress successfully.

5.1.2.2 Micro-mineral supplementation

5.1.2.2.1 Zinc

Zn is a "member" of the antioxidant network because it is a cofactor of a very important antioxidant enzyme: Cu/Zn-SOD. Zinc plays a role in depressing the free radicals and inhibiting lipid peroxidation and GSH depletion. Zn can have direct antioxidant function and it is necessary for the prevention of free radical formation. However, it does not act directly against them [53]. Zinc supplementation has positive effects on antioxidant status of birds [61–63]. Zinc may play an important role in suppressing free radicals because it works as a cofactor (Cu/Zn-SOD) and inhibits NADPH-dependent lipid peroxidation [64], thus improving antioxidant status: increased serum Vitamin C and E concentrations [65] and decreased MDA levels [57, 66] (**Table 3**, [56]).

5.1.2.2.2 Selenium

Organoselenium compounds are essential micronutrients and are required for cellular defense against oxidative stress and optimal immune function. Selenium is necessary for cellular function and is a component of antioxidant enzymes: an important part (cofactor) of GPx, which works as an important antioxidant enzyme, protecting cells against free radical damage and oxidative stress [53]. Selenium supplementation improved antioxidant status in poultry under heat stress [51, 55, 58]. It is suggested that the metabolic role of Se is to protect cells against oxidation and tissue damage. Rapid oxidation of GSH to GSSH is necessary to compensate the heat stress caused ROS production. However, Se supplementation increases the level of available NADPH to promote the activation of GR, leading to increased GSSH reduction to GSH [67]. Therefore, Se supplementation affected GPx activity and the GPx/GSH ratio (**Table 3**).

Results of studies done with separated supplementation of Vitamin A (9000–15000 IU/kg diet), Vitamin E (150–500 mg/kg diet), Vitamin C (150–500 mg/kg diet), Zn (30 or 60 mg/kg diet) and Se (0,1-1 mg/kg diet), show that antioxidant status improved in poultry under heat stress. Antioxidant potential has been reported to be more efficient and important in combination than single antioxidant nutrients [68]. The latest research studies show that interactions between vitamin-vitamin and vitamin-minerals used in combination have more improved effects on

Author(s)	Spices	Duration of the study	Environmental temperature	Amount of supplementation (mg/kg diet)	Other effects
Sahin et al. [65]	Japanese quail	10–42 day	34°C (8 h/day)	Zn:30 or 60 mg/kg diet	↑Vitamin C concentration in serum ↓ MDA
Kucuk et al. [57]	broiler	1–42 day	34°C (24 h/day)	Zn: 30 mg/kg diet	↓MDA
Kucuk, [66]	Japanese quail	10–40day	35°C (8 h/day)	Zn: 30 mg/kg diet	↓ MDA
Harsini et al. [55]	broiler	1–49 day	37°C (8 h/day)	Se: 1 mg/kg diet	⦰Zn concentration ↑GPx
Mahmound and Edens, [58]	broiler	1–28 day	33°C (24 h/day for 4 weeks)	Se: 0.46 ppm/ kg diet	↑GSH, GSSG, GPx, GPx/GR ratio
Sahin et al. [51]	Japanese quail	10–40 day	34°C (24 h/day)	Se: 0.1 / 0.2 mg/kg diet	↑serum Vitamin E, A, Zn ↓ MDA

GPx = glutathione peroxidase concentration in blood; GR = glutathione reductase concentration in blood; GSH = reduced glutathione concentration in blood; GSSG = glutathione disulphide concentration in blood; GPx = glutathione peroxidase concentration in blood; MDA = malondialdehyde concentration in blood; Se = selenium; Zn = zinc.
↑ Increase; ↓ decrease; ⦰ no effect.

Table 3.
Effects of micro mineral supplementation under heat stress based on different studies [56].

Supplementation	Author(s)	Spices	Duration of the study	Environmental temperature	Amount of supplementation	Other effects
Vitamin C + Zn	Naila et al. 2014	broiler	22-42d	40 °C (12 h/day)	300 mg Vit. C + 60 mg Zn	↓mortality
Vitamin A+ Zn	Kucuk et al. [57]	broiler	1-42d	34°C (24 h/day)	15 000 IU Vit A + 30 mg	↓MDA
Vitamin E+ Se	Harsini et al. [55]	broiler	1-49d	37°C (8 h/day)	0.5 mg Se + 152 mg Vit.E	↓MDA ↑SOD

MDA = malondialdehyde concentration in blood; SOD = superoxide dismutase concentration in blood, Se = selenium, Zn = zinc.
↑ Increase; ↓ decrease.

Table 4.
Effects of vitamin and mineral interactions under heat stress based on different studies [56].

the antioxidant status and performance of poultry under heat stress than they do separately. Literature data on combinations of vitamin and mineral supplementation can be seen in **Table 4** [56].

5.1.2.3 Plant extracts

Dried oregano powder (0.5% and 1%) can be supplemented for ducks. Oregano (*Origanum vulgare* L.) is an herb extract used as an additive in poultry nutrition. It is an aromatic plant, containing more than 30 phenolic antioxidants constituents, including also anti-inflammatory and anti-microbial activity. It can also have beneficial effects on production, mortality, microflora, and the immune system [69]. Antioxidant enzyme activity (SOD, GPx) was improved in poultry [69]. These results suggest that dried oregano powder addition could decrease the changes in antioxidant enzymes under heat stress.

5.1.2.4 Probiotics

Probiotics are non-digestive alternative growth promoters used in poultry nutrition. Probiotics can improve animal performance, and it can manipulate and maintain beneficial microflora in the gut. Several studies prove that probiotics supplementation to feed improves production parameters in poultry [70, 71]. Supplementation of probiotics (*Bacillus Subtilis*: 1x108 CFU/kg feed) decreased MDA activity and uric acid concentration, and also improved antioxidant response in ducks [72, 73].

6. The effect of heat stress on the performance of broilers reduced by using feed additives

6.1 The effect of heat stress on the performance of broilers

After reviewing the relevant research, we identified three different types of heat stress (HS) that have been applied in experiments: acute, cyclic and chronic. In the case of acute HS, the elevated temperature lasts from several hours up to 24 hours. After exposure to HS, sample and data collection occurs. This type of arrangement is suitable to study the immediate effect of heat stress. However, in temperate countries, even in the case of cooled stables, the actual barn temperature shows a daily cycle which can be mimicked by the cyclic HS environment (4–10 hours per day in the range of three days per week to daily up to 10 days long). In tropical countries, this kind of fluctuation is much less pronounced. Therefore, the environmental conditions can be best modeled with a chronic HS (continuous HS environment usually during the second half of fattening) model [74].

The most often claimed effect of heat stress is a reduction of feed intake. As an immediate effect, acute heat stress reduces feed intake by about 25% (**Table 5**).

Applying the heat stress repeatedly but allowing regeneration at thermoneutral (TN) temperature (cyclic HS-simulating the day-night temperature fluctuation) results in an adaptation, as during this period the lowest decline (in between 5 and 15%) in performance data (feed intake, daily gain and feed conversion ratio) can be observed (**Table 5**). Chronic heat stress will approximately double the negative effect compared to cyclic heat stress (7–11% point), but still some adaptation can be seen compared to acute heat stress. Acute HS has a dramatic effect on daily gain, as even negative values (weight loss) can occur, which makes it impracticable to calculate the feed conversion ratio. Therefore, researchers did not publish such data. The nutrient content of the unconsumed feed itself does not justify the negative energy balance; therefore, one can assume that the energy and nutrient needs of the HS response are high. When adaptation can occur; cyclic HS has a less adverse effect than chronic HS on both daily gain and the feed conversion ratio (**Table 5**).

6.2 Mitigation capacity of various feed additives on HS in broilers

One long term aim of researchers is to be able to mitigate the negative effects of heat stress. Supplementation of effective feed additives could be useful for improving intestinal absorption and minimizing the adverse effects of HS [92]. To have

Thermo-neutral temperature, °C	Heat stress temperature, °C	HS period, day of life	HS type	Feed intake, g/day			Average daily gain, g/day			Feed conversion ratio, kg/kg			Source
				Treatment		Change to TN %[c]	Treatment		Change to TN %[c]	Treatment		Change to TN %[c]	
				TN[a]	HS[b]		TN	HS		TN	HS		
18–19	38	20,41	acute[d]	115.2 ± 32.1	79.5 ± 16.2	−26.5 ± 24.7	78.5 ± 13.0	−1.3 ± 45.7	−102.9 ± 55.4				[75, 76]
20–28	31–36.2	15–49	cyclic[e]	125.8 ± 44.8	114.7 ± 33.6	−7.2 ± 9.0	69.4 ± 17.9	57.8 ± 13.7	−15.4 ± 12.8	1.95 ± 0.32	2.15 ± 0.54	9.1 ± 14.26	[77–84]
20–26	27.8–35	1–42	chronic[f]	132.8 ± 42.0	112.7 ± 33.5	−14.4 ± 10.0	70.5 ± 14.2	51.5 ± 11.5	−26.3 ± 14.0	1.85 ± 0.27	2.17 ± 0.33	18.1 ± 10.2	[81, 85–91]

[a]*Thermoneutral environment.*
[b]*Heat stress environment.*
[c]*(TN-HS)/TN*100, average values of the calculations from the research cited.*
[d]*HS environment from several hours to 24 hours.*
[e]*HS environment 4–10 hours per day in the range of three days per week to daily up to 10 days.*
[f]*Continuous HS environment (24 hours/day) usually during the second half of the fattening.*

Table 5.
Effect of heat stress on the growth performance of broilers (means ± s.d.).

TNt[a], °C	HSt[b], °C	HS period, days of life	HS type	Dietary treatment	Treatment type	Concentration of feed additives in the diet	Feed intake, g/day				Source
							TN[c]	HS[d]	HS + treatment[e]	Mitigation[f] %	
22	32	1–42	chronic[g]	betaine + vit E	combined[l]	1.2 g/kg + 500 mg/kg	111.1	78.5	83.3	14.7	[85]
22	32	1–42	chronic	Cr + vit C	combined	1.2 mg/kg + 500 mg/kg	111.1	78.5	83.1	14.1	[85]
22	32	1–42	chronic	cumin + tumeric	combined	1% + 1%	111.1	78.5	87.9	28.8	[85]
22	32	1–42	chronic	KCl + Na bicarbonate	combined	1.5 + 2 g/kg	111.1	78.5	83.1	14.1	[85]
22	32	1–42	chronic	propolis + vit A	combined	1 g/kg +15000 IU/kg	111.1	78.5	84.3	17.8	[85]
26	35	26–42	chronic	MOS + probiotic [i]	combined	0.5% + 0.1%	76.5	64.0	62.4	−12.8	[87]
	32	22–42	chronic	fumaric acid	single[m]	5 g/kg	160.7	142.4	143.4	5.7	[86]
23	32	22–42	chronic	fumaric acid	single	10 g/kg	160.7	142.4	138.7	−20.0	[86]
23	32	22–42	chronic	fumaric acid	single	15 g/kg	160.7	142.4	148.6	33.8	[86]
26	35	26–42	chronic	MOS	single	0.5%	76.5	64.0	63.3	−5.6	[87]
24	35	15–35	chronic	probiotic [j]	single	0.1%	86.1	82.0	85.6	87.8	[88]
26	35	26–42	chronic	probiotic [i]	single	0.1%	76.5	64.0	65.9	15.2	[87]
25	36	25–42	cyclic[h]	vit E + vit C	combined	100 mg/kg + 200 mg/kg	78.2	73.6	74.6	21.7	[78]
25	36	25–42	cyclic	vit E + vit C+ probiotic [k]	combined	100 mg/kg +200 mg/kg + 2 g/kg	78.2	73.6	74.4	17.4	[78]
25	36	25–42	cyclic	probiotic	single	2 g/kg	78.2	73.6	73.5	−2.2	[78]
25	36	25–42	cyclic	vit C	single	200 mg/kg	78.2	73.6	74.8	26.1	[78]
25	36	25–42	cyclic	vit E	single	100 mg/kg	78.2	73.6	73.5	−2.2	[78]
24	34	15–35	cyclic	vit E	single	150 mg/kg	99.5	91.9	89.2	−35.2	[79]
24	34	15–35	cyclic	vit E	single	150 mg/kg	104.1	87.1	89.3	13.0	[79]
			chronic		combined				Average ± sd	*12.8 ± 13.7*	

TNt[a], °C	HSt[b], °C	HS period, days of life	HS type	Dietary treatment	Treatment type	Concentration of feed additives in the diet	Feed intake, g/day				Source
							TN[c]	HS[d]	HS + treatment[e]	Mitigation[f] %	
			chronic		single				Average ± sd	*19.5 ± 38.1*	
			chronic		overall[n]				Average ± sd	16.1 ± 27.6	
			cyclic		combined				Average ± sd	*19.6 ± 3.1*	
			cyclic		single				Average ± sd	*−0.1 ± 22.9*	
			cyclic		overall				Average ± sd	5.5 ± 21.1	

[a]*Thermoneutral temperature.*
[b]*Heat stress temperature.*
[c]*Thermoneutral environment, control feed.*
[d]*Heat stress environment, control feed.*
[e]*Heat stress environment and specialty feed supplement fortified diet.*
[f]*% mitigation = (HS treatment - HS control)/(TN control – HS control) x 100.*
[g]*HS environment 4–10 hours per day in the range of three days per week to daily up to 10 days.*
[h]*Continuous HS environment (24 hours/day) usually during the second half of the fattening.*
[i]Lactobacillus plantarum, Lactobacillus delbrueckii *ssp. Bulgaricus,* Lactobacillus acidophilus, Lactobacillus rhamnosus, Bifidobacterium bifidum, *and* Streptococcus salivarius *ssp. Thermophilus and* Enterococcus faecium.
[j]Lactobacillus pentosus *ITA23 and* Lactobacillus acidophilus *ITA44.*
[k]Saccharomyces cerevisiae *and* Lactobacillus acidophilus.
[l]*Combination of two or more feed additives are used.*
[m]*Only one feed additive used.*
[n]*HS type averages regardless of single or combined supplementation.*

Table 6.
Mitigation capacity of various feed additives on HS in broilers' growth performance (daily feed intake, g/day).

TNt[a], °C	HSt[b], °C	HS period, days of life	HS type	Dietary treatment	Treatment type	Concentration of feed additives in the diet	Average daily gain, g/day				Source
							TN[c]	HS[d]	HS + treatment[e]	Mitigation[f] %	
22	32	1–42	chronic[g]	betaine + vit E	combined[l]	1.2 g/kg + 500 mg/kg	62.0	33.9	42.0	28.8	[85]
22	32	1–42	chronic	Cr + vit C	combined	1.2 mg/kg + 500 mg/kg	62.0	33.9	41.6	27.4	[85]
22	32	1–42	chronic	cumin+tumeric	combined	1% + 1%	62.0	33.9	41.0	25.3	[85]
22	32	1–42	chronic	KCl + Na bicarbonate	combined	1.5 g/kg +2 g/kg	62.0	33.9	40.9	24.9	[85]
22	32	1–42	chronic	propolis + vit A	combined	1 g/kg +15000 IU/kg	62.0	33.9	41.1	25.6	[85]
26	35	26–42	chronic	MOS + probiotic [i]	combined	0,5% + 0,1%	57.4	38.7	41.5	15.0	[87]
23	32	22–42	chronic	fumaric acid	single[m]	5 g/kg	83.3	61.4	68.6	32.6	[86]
23	32	22–42	chronic	fumaric acid	single	10 g/kg	86.3	61.4	69.1	30.6	[86]
23	32	22–42	chronic	fumaric acid	single	15 g/kg	83.3	61.4	76.2	67.5	[86]
26	35	26–42	chronic	MOS	single	0,50%	57.4	38.7	45.4	35.8	[87]
24	35	15–35	chronic	probiotic [j]	single	0,10%	53.8	43.3	48.0	44.8	[88]
26	35	26–42	chronic	probiotic [i]	single	0,10%	57.4	38.7	41.1	12.8	[87]
25	36	25–42	cyclic[h]	vit E + vit C	combined	100 mg/kg + 200 mg/kg	43.6	38.6	41.2	52.0	[78]
25	36	25–42	cyclic	vit E + vit C + probiotic [g]	combined	100 mg/kg +200 mg/kg + 2 g/kg	43.6	38.6	42.7	82.0	[78]
25	36	25–42	cyclic	probiotic [k]	single	2 g/kg	43.6	38.6	41.3	54.0	[78]
25	36	25–42	cyclic	vit C	single	200 mg/kg	43.6	38.6	40.1	30.0	[78]
25	36	25–42	cyclic	vit E	single	100 mg/kg	43.6	38.6	39.8	24.0	[78]
24	34	15–35	cyclic	vit E	single	150 mg/kg	55.7	46.4	48.5	23.1	[79]
24	34	15–35	cyclic	vit E	single	150 mg/kg	54.0	48.7	48.4	−4.7	[79]
			chronic		combined				Average ± sd	*24.5 ± 4.9*	

TNt[a], °C	HSt[b], °C	HS period, days of life	HS type	Dietary treatment	Treatment type	Concentration of feed additives in the diet	Average daily gain, g/day				Source
							TN[c]	HS[d]	HS + treatment[e]	Mitigation[f] %	
			chronic		single				Average ± sd	*37.4 ± 18.1*	
			chronic		overall[n]				Average ± sd	30.9 ± 14.3	
			cyclic		combined				Average ± sd	*67.0 ± 21.2*	
			cyclic		single				Average ± sd	*25.3 ± 20.9*	
			cyclic		overall				Average ± sd	37.2 ± 27.9	

[a]*Thermoneutral temperature.*
[b]*Heat stress temperature.*
[c]*Thermoneutral environment, control feed.*
[d]*Heat stress environment, control feed.*
[e]*Heat stress environment and specialty feed supplement fortified diet.*
[f]*% mitigation = (HS treatment - HS control)/(TN control – HS control) x 100.*
[g]*HS environment 4–10 hours per day in the range of three days per week to daily up to 10 days.*
[h]*Continuous HS environment (24 hours/day) usually during the second half of the fattening.*
[i]Lactobacillus plantarum, Lactobacillus delbrueckii *ssp. Bulgaricus,* Lactobacillus acidophilus, Lactobacillus rhamnosus, Bifidobacterium bifidum, *and* Streptococcus salivarius *ssp. Thermophilus and* Enterococcus faecium.
[j]Lactobacillus pentosus *ITA23 and* Lactobacillus acidophilus *ITA44.*
[k]Saccharomyces cerevisiae *and* Lactobacillus acidophilus.
[l]*Combination of two or more feed additives are used.*
[m]*Only one feed additive used.*
[n]*HS type averages regardless of single or combined supplementation.*

Table 7.
Mitigation capacity of various feed additives on HS in broilers' growth performance (average daily gain, g/day).

TNt[a], °C	HSt[b], °C	HS period, days of life	HS type	Dietary treatment	Treatment type	Concentration of feed additives in the diet	Feed conversion ratio, kg/kg				Source
							TN[c]	HS[d]	HS + treatment[e]	Mitigation[f]%	
22	32	1–42	chronic[g]	betaine + vit E	combined[l]	1.2 g/kg + 500 mg/kg	1.8	2.3	2.0	64.2	[85]
22	32	1–42	chronic	Cr + vit C	combined	1.2 mg/kg + 500 mg/kg	1.8	2.3	2.0	62.3	[85]
22	32	1–42	chronic	cumin + tumeric	combined	1% + 1%	1.8	2.3	2.1	34.0	[85]
22	32	1–42	chronic	KCl + Na bicarbonate	combined	1.5 g/kg + 2 g/kg	1.8	2.3	2.0	54.7	[85]
22	32	1–42	chronic	propolis + vit A	combined	1 g/kg + 15000 IU/kg	1.8	2.3	2.0	52.8	[85]
26	35	26–42	chronic	MOS + probiotic [i]	combined	0.5% + 0.1%	1.3	1.7	1.5	50.0	[87]
23	32	22–42	chronic	fumaric acid	single[m]	5 g/kg	1.9	2.3	2.1	59.0	[86]
23	32	22–42	chronic	fumaric acid	single	10 g/kg	1.9	2.3	2.0	82.1	[86]
23	32	22–42	chronic	fumaric acid	single	15 g/kg	1.9	2.3	2.0	94.9	[86]
26	35	26–42	chronic	MOS	single	0.5%	1.3	1.7	1.4	82.4	[87]
24	35	15–35	chronic	probiotic [j]	single	0.1%	1.6	1.9	1.8	34.5	[88]
26	35	26–42	chronic	probiotic [i]	single	0.1%	1.3	1.7	1.6	20.6	[87]
25	36	25–42	cyclic[h]	vit E + vit C	combined	100 mg/kg + 200 mg/kg	1.8	1.9	1.8	81.8	[78]
25	36	25–42	cyclic	vit E + vit C+ probiotic[k]	combined	100 mg/kg +200 mg/kg + 2 g/kg	1.8	1.9	1.7	145.5	[78]
25	36	25–42	cyclic	probiotic	single	2 g/kg	1.8	1.9	1.8	109.1	[78]
25	36	25–42	cyclic	vit C	single	200 mg/kg	1.8	1.9	1.9	27.3	[78]
25	36	25–42	cyclic	vit E	single	100 mg/kg	1.8	1.9	1.9	45.5	[78]
24	34	15–35	cyclic	vit E	single	150 mg/kg	1.8	2.0	1.8	73.5	[79]
24	34	15–35	cyclic	vit E	single	150 mg/kg	1.9	1.8	1.8	40.1	[79]
			chronic		combined				Average ± sd	*53.0 ± 10.8*	
			chronic		single				Average ± sd	*62.2 ± 29.6*	

TNt[a], °C	HSt[b], °C	HS period, days of life	HS type	Dietary treatment	Treatment type	Concentration of feed additives in the diet	Feed conversion ratio, kg/kg				Source
							TN[c]	HS[d]	HS + treatment[e]	Mitigation[f]%	
			chronic		overall[n]				Average ± sd	57.6 ± 21.8	
			cyclic		combined				Average ± sd	*113.6 ± 45.0*	
			cyclic		single				Average ± sd	*59.1 ± 32.7*	
			cyclic		overall				Average ± sd	74.7 ± 41.9	

[a]*Thermoneutral temperature.*
[b]*Heat stress temperature.*
[c]*Thermoneutral environment, control feed.*
[d]*Heat stress environment, control feed.*
[e]*Heat stress environment and specialty feed supplement fortified diet.*
[f]*% mitigation = (HS treatment - HS control)/(TN control – HS control) x 100.*
[g]*HS environment 4–10 hours per day in the range of three days per week to daily up to 10 days.*
[h]*Continuous HS environment (24 hours/day) usually during the second half of the fattening.*
[i]Lactobacillus plantarum, Lactobacillus delbrueckii *ssp. Bulgaricus,* Lactobacillus acidophilus, Lactobacillus rhamnosus, Bifidobacterium bifidum, *and* Streptococcus salivarius *ssp. Thermophilus and* Enterococcus faecium.
[j]Lactobacillus pentosus *ITA23 and* Lactobacillus acidophilus *ITA44.*
[k]Saccharomyces cerevisiae *and* Lactobacillus acidophilus.
[l]*Combination of two or more feed additives are used.*
[m]*Only one feed additive used.*
[n]*HS type averages regardless of single or combined supplementation.*

Table 8.
Mitigation capacity of various feed additives on HS in broilers' growth performance (feed conversion ratio, kg/kg).

more clear information on effectiveness of various feed supplements Ortega and Szabó [93] suggested the calculation of mitigation capacity (see subsection 2 in the present chapter). However, researchers [93] also point out that contrary to the numerous publications in the field, only a limited number of studies are suitable for using this calculation, as it requires at least three treatment groups. HS effect mitigating supplements are usually vitamins expressing antioxidant capacity, probiotics and plant extracts (**Tables 6–8**).

It can be seen that - overall - the most difficult parameter to improve is that of feed intake (**Table 7**), as the feed additives studied have quite variable mitigation capacities. The overall mitigation percentage is only about 5–15%.Bettervalueswere obtained in the case of chronic heat stress compared to cyclic heat stress, but different feed additives were used. The highest improvement (above 85%) was achieved with a probiotic [88]. However, other probiotics were much less effective.

The adversely affected daily gain can be improved by about 30–35%, and the feed conversion ratio increased up to 60–70%. Observing the mitigation capacity of different feed additives in this regard, it seems that probiotics and vitamins can be the most effective mitigators, especially when they are applied in combination [84]. However, further research is needed to determine the most effective microbe combination(s), and the most effective levels of vitamins, as well as their interactive effects. Only one study reported results with fumaric acid supplementation which also seems promising, but more research is still needed [86]. Quite a few authors have tested the feed supplements in combination, which is in line with feed industry trends. Therefore, we calculated the average % mitigation value for combined and single applications. Data shows that combined applications are more effective in cyclic heat stress conditions, while that benefit cannot be observed in chronic heat stress.

7. Conclusions

Based on the scientific findings presented in this chapter, the following important conclusions can be drawn:

- Using fat in the diet (up to 5%) can reduce heat production in livestock.

- Vitamins (e.g. A, E and C) are capable of reacting with free radicals, thereby reducing their amounts and lipid peroxidation in the poultry. However, micro minerals (e.g. Zn, Se) are not directly capable of preventing or reducing ROS-formation, but they are essential cofactors for those enzymes which are reacting with free radicals.

- Vitamin E and Vitamin C supplementation improved antioxidant parameters (CAT, GR, GSH, MDA, SOD) due to their essential antioxidant function. Both Zn and Se are also improving antioxidant parameters (GR, GSH, GPx, and MDA).

- Antioxidant potential of vitamins and micro minerals is more efficient in combination under heat stress in poultry nutrition.

- Plant extracts (e.g. oregano) could decrease the negative effects of heat stress on antioxidant enzyme activity due its antioxidant constituents.

- Betaine reduces heat production in animals at high ambient temperatures.

- Acute heat stress induced a drop in feed intake and increased nutrient demand will result even in weight loss. However, if heat stress is prolonged, adaptation will occur.

- Probiotics and vitamins (C and E) seem to be the most effective means of reducing the negative effects of heat stress.

- Main conclusion for the practice: Different feed additives and supplementation strategies (single vs. combined) can be more effective in temperate and tropical countries. Therefore, in order to decide which feed additive to use and in what form (single or combined) the most effectively, it is recommended that farmers carry out a pre-study in the given climatic and feeding conditions.

Author details

László Babinszky*, Csaba Szabó and Márta Horváth
Department of Animal Nutrition and Physiology, University of Debrecen, Debrecen, Hungary

*Address all correspondence to: babinszky@agr.unideb.hu

References

[1] Thornton, P.K., J.van de Steeg, A. Notenbaert, M. Herrero. 2009. The impacts of climate change on livestock and livestock systems in developing countries: a review of what we know and what we need to know. Agricultural Systems. 101: 113–127.

[2] Nardone, A., B. Ronchi, N. Lacetera, M.S. Ranieri, and U. Bernabucci. 2010. Effects of climate changes on animal production and sustainability of livestock systems. Livestock Science. 130: 57–69.

[3] Summer, A., I. Lora, P. Formaggioni, F. Gottardo. 2019. Impact of heat stress on milk and meat production. Animal Frontiers. 1: 39–46.

[4] USDA. 2021. United States Department of Agriculture. Foreign Agricultural Service/ Global Market Analysis. Report. July 12, 2021.

[5] FAO. 2020. Food and Agriculture Organization of the United Nations, Emerging trends and outlook, FAO Report, December 2020.

[6] Daghir, N. J. 2009. Nutritional strategies to reduce heat stress in broilers and broiler breeders. Lohmann Information. 1: 6-15.

[7] Lin, H., H. C. Jiao, J. Buyse, E. Decuypere. 2006. Strategies for preventing heat stress in poultry. World's Poultry Science Journal. 1: 71-86.

[8] Wolfenson, D., D. Bachrach, M. Maman, Y. Graber, I. Rozenboim. 2001. Evaporative cooling of ventral regions of the skin in heat-stressed laying hens. Poultry Science. 7: 958-964.

[9] Babinszky L., V. Halas, M.W.A. Verstegen. 2011. Impacts of climate change on animal production and quality of animal food products (Chapter 10) In: J. A. Blanco and H. Kheradmand (Eds): Climate change, socioeconomic effects. InTech Publisher. London, UK. 165-190.

[10] Babinszky, L., M. Horváth, J. Remenyik, M.W.A. Verstegen. 2019. The adverse effects of heat stress on the antioxidant status and performance of pigs and poultry and reducing these effects with nutritional tools. In: Wouter H. Hendriks, Martin W. A. Verstegen, László Babinszky. Poultry and pig nutrition. Challenges of the 21st century. Wageningen, Wageningen Academic Publishers. 187- 208.

[11] FASS (Federation of Animal Science Societies). 2010. Guide for the care and use of agricultural animals in research and teaching, (January 2010), ISBN: 978–1–884706-11- 0, Champaign, Illinois, USA. www.fass.org/docs/agguide3rd/Ag_Guide_3rd_ed.pdf

[12] DEFRA (Department for Environment, Food and Rural Affairs). 2005. Heat stress in poultry, solving the problem. UK. Nobel House 17 Smith Square London SW1P 3JR. www.defra.gov.uk

[13] Dawson, W. R., G. C. Whittow. 2000. Regulation of body temperature (Chapter 14). In: G. C. Whittow (Ed). Sturkie's avian physiology. Academic Press, San Diego, CA.USA. 390–685.

[14] Abbas, A., M. J. Khan, M. Naeem, M. Ayaz, A. Sufyan, M. H. Somro. 2012. Cation anion balance in avian diet: A review. Agricultural Science Research Journal. 2: 302-307.

[15] Toyomizu, M., M. Tokuda, A. Mujahid, Y. Akiba. 2005. Progressive alteration to core temperature, respiration and blood acid-base balance in broiler chickens exposed to acute heat stress. Journal of Poultry Science. 42: 110-118.

[16] Saeed, M., G. Abbas, M. Alagawany, A. A. Kamboh, M. E. A. El-Hack, A. F. Khafagaf, S. Chao. 2019. Heat stress management in poultry farms: A comprehensive overview. Journal of Thermal Biology. 84: 414–425.

[17] EW-Nutrition. 2020. Heat stress in poultry. https://ew-nutrition.com/heat-stress-in-poultry/

[18] Mustaf, S.; Kahraman, N.S.; Firat, M.Z. 2009. Intermittent partial surface wetting and its effect on body-surface temperatures and egg production of white brown domestic laying hens in Antalya (Turkey). British Poultry Science. 50: 33–38.

[19] Fedde, M.R. 1998. Relationship of structure and function of the avian respiratory system to disease susceptibility. Poultry Science. 77: 1130–1138.

[20] Lucas J., M. H. Rostagno. 2013. Impact of heat stress on poultry production. Animals. 3: 356-369.

[21] Syafwan, S., R. P. Kwakkel, M.W.A. Verstegen. 2011. Heat stress and feeding strategies in meattype chickens. World's Poultry Science Journal. 67: 653-673.

[22] Havenstein, G.B., P. R. Ferket, M.A. Qureshi. 2003. Growth, livability, and feed conversion of 1957 versus 2001 broilers when fed representative 1957 and 2001 broiler diets. Poultry Science. 82: 1500- 1508.

[23] Babinszky, L. 1998. Dietary fat and milk production (Chapter 8). In: The lactating sow, M.W. A. Verstegen, P.J. Moughan and J. W. Schrama (Eds). Wageningen Pers. The Netherlands. 143-157.

[24] Das, S., T. K. Palai, S. R. Mishra, D. Das, B. Jena.2011. Nutrition in relation to diseases and heat stress in poultry. A review. Veterinary World. 9: 429-432.

[25] Musharaf, N. A., J. D. Latshaw. 1999. Heat increment as affected by protein and amino acid nutrition. World's Poultry Science Journal. 55: 233–240.

[26] Mateos, G.G., J. L. Sell, J. A. Eastwood. 1982. Rate of food passage (transit time) as influenced by level of supplemental fat. Poultry Science. 61: 94–100.

[27] Mateos, G.G., J. L. Sell. 1981. Influence of fat and carbohydrate source on rate of food passage of semi-purified diets for laying hens. Poultry Science. 60: 2114–2119.

[28] Attia, Y.A., M. A. Al-Harthi, Sh Elnaggar. 2018. A. Productive, physiological and immunological responses of two broiler strains fed different dietary regimens and exposed to heat stress. Italian Journal of Animal Science. 17: 686–697

[29] Ghazalah, A.A., M.O. Abd-Elsamee, A.M. Ali. 2008. Influence of dietary energy and poultry fat on the response of broiler chicks to heat therm. International Journal of Poultry Science. 7: 355-359.

[30] Abdel-Moneim, A.-M.E., A. M. Shehata, R. E. Khidr, V. K. Paswan, N. S. Ibrahim, A. A. El-Ghoul, S. A. Aldhumri, S. A. Gabr, N. M. Mesalam, A. M. Elbaz, M. A. Elsayed, M. M. Wakwak, T. A. Ebeid. 2021. Nutritional manipulation to combat heat stress in poultry – A comprehensive review. Journal of Thermal Biology. https://doi.org/10.1016/j.jtherbio.2021.102915

[31] Barzegar, S., S. B. Wu, M. Choct, R. A. Swick. 2020. Factors affecting energy metabolism and evaluating net energy of poultry feed. Poultry Science. 99:.487–498.

[32] McDonald, P., R. A. Edwards, J. F. D. Greenhalgh, C. A. Morgan, L. A. Sinclair, R. G. Wilkinson. 2011. Animal calorimetry: methods for measuring

heat production and energy retention (Chapter 11.3). In: Animal nutrition. Pearson Publisher. Seventh Edition. UK. 262-270.

[33] McKee, J. S., P. C. Harrison, G. L. Riskowski. 1997. Effects of supplemental ascorbic acid on the energy conversion of broiler chicks during heat stress and feed withdrawal. Poultry Science. 76: 1278–1286.

[34] Abdelsattar, M.M., M. N. Abd El-Ati, A.M. Hussein, A.M. Saleem. 2019. Impact of betaine as a feed additive on livestock performance, carcass characteristics and meat quality: A review. SVU-International Journal of Agricultural Science. 2: 33-42.

[35] Eklund, M., E. Bauer, J. Wamatu, R. Mosenthin. 2005. Potential nutritional and physiological functions of betaine in livestock. Nutrition Research Reviews. 18: 31–48

[36] Ahmed, M. M.N., Z. S. H. Ismail, A. A. A. Abdel-Wareth. 2018. Application of betaine as feed additives in poultry nutrition: A review. Journal of Experimental and Applied Animal Sciences. 3: 266-272.

[37] Arumugam, M.K.; M. C. Paal Jr. T. M. Donohue, M. Ganesan, N. A. Osna, K. K. Kharbanda. 2021. Beneficial effects of betaine: A comprehensive review. Biology. 10: 456. https://doi.org/10.3390/biology10060456

[38] Saeed, M., D. Babazadeh, M. Naveed, M. A. Arain, F. U. Hassan, S. Chao. 2017. Reconsidering betaine as a natural anti-heat stress agent in poultry industry: A review. Tropical Animal Health and Production. 49: 1329–1338.

[39] Wasti, S. N. Sah, B. Mishra. 2020. Impact of heat stress on poultry health and performances, and potential mitigation strategies. Animals. 10(8), 1266; https://doi.org/10.3390/ani10081266

[40] Schrama, J. W., M.J. W Heetkamp,. P.H. Simmins, W. J. J. Gerrits. 2003. Dietary betaine supplementation affects energy metabolism of pigs. Journal of Animal Science. 81: 1202-1209.

[41] Altan, Ö., A. Pabuçcuoğlu, A. Altan, S. Konyalioğlu, H. Bayraktar. 2003. Effect of heat stress on oxidative stress, lipid peroxidation and some stress parameters in broilers. British Poultry Science. 4: 545-550.

[42] Costantini, D., S. Verhulst. 2009. Does high antioxidant capacity indicate low oxidative stress? Functional Ecology. 3: 506-509.

[43] Lara, L., M. Rostagno. 2013. Impact of heat stress on poultry production. Animals. 2: 356-369.

[44] Yang, L., G. Y. Tan, Y. Q. Fu, J. H. Feng, M. H. Zhang. 2010. Effects of acute heat stress and subsequent stress removal on function of hepatic mitochondrial respiration, ROS production and lipid peroxidation in broiler chickens. Comparative Biochemistry and Physiology Part C: Toxicology and Pharmacology. 2: 204-208.

[45] Akbarian, A., A. Golian, H. Kermanshahi, S. De Smet, J. Michiels. 2015. Antioxidant enzyme activities, plasma hormone levels and serum metabolites of finishing broiler chickens reared under high ambient temperature and fed lemon and orange peel extracts and Curcuma xanthorrhiza essential oil. Journal of Animal Physiology and Animal Nutrition. 1: 150-162.

[46] Kutlu, H. R., J. M. Forbes. 1993. Changes in growth and blood parameters in heat-stressed broiler chicks in response to dietary ascorbic acid. Livestock Production Science. 4: 335-350.

[47] Anderson, R. A. 1994. Stress effects on chromium nutrition of humans and

farm animals. In: Lyons TP, Jacques KA, editors. Biotechnology in Feed Industry. Nottingham, England: University Press. 267–274.

[48] Zeng, T., J.J. Li, D.Q. Wang, G.Q. Li, G.L. Wang, L.Z. Lu. 2014. Effects of heat stress on antioxidant defence system, inflammatory injury, and heat shock proteins of Muscovy and Pekin ducks: evidence for differential thermal sensitivities. Cell Stress Chaperones. 6: 895-901. DOI: 10.1007/s12192-014-0514-7.

[49] Zeng, T., X. Jiang, J. Li, D. Wang, G. Li, L. Lu, G. Wang. 2013. Comparative proteomic analysis of the hepatic response to heat stress in Muscovy and Pekin ducks: insight into thermal tolerance related to energy metabolism. Plos One, 10: e76917. pp. 1-17. DOI: 10.1371/journal.pone.0076917.

[50] Tan, G. Y.,L. Yang, Y.Q. Fu, J.H. Feng, M.H. Zhang. 2010. Effects of different acute high ambient temperatures on function of hepatic mitochondrial respiration, antioxidative enzymes, and oxidative injury in broiler chickens. Poultry Science. 1: 115-122.

[51] Sahin, K., N. Sahin, M. Sari, M.F. Gursu. 2002. Effects of vitamins E and A supplementation on lipid peroxidation and concentration of some mineral in broilers reared under heat stress (32°C), Nutritional Research. 22: 723–731.

[52] Khan, R., S. Naz, Z. Nikousefat, M. Selvaggi, V. Laudadio, V. Tufarelli. 2012. Effect of ascorbic acid in heat-stressed poultry. World's Poultry Science Journal. 3: 477-490.

[53] Horváth, M. 2021. Alleviating the adverse effect of chronic heat stress on selected antioxidant parameters and performance of meat type ducks by dietary vitamin E, vitamin C, selenium and zinc supplementation. PhD Thesis. University of Debrecen, Hungary.

[54] Maini, S., S.K. Rastogi, J.P. Korde, A.K. Madan, S.K. Shukla. 2007. Evaluation of oxidative stress and its amelioration through certain antioxidants in broilers during summer. The Journal of Poultry Science. 3: 339-347.

[55] Harsini, S. G., M. Habibiyan, M. M. Moeini, A. R. Abdolmohammadi. 2012. Effects of dietary selenium, vitamin E, and their combination on growth, serum metabolites, and antioxidant defense system in skeletal muscle of broilers under heat stress. Biological Trace Element Research. 3: 322-330.

[56] Horváth, M., L. Babinszky. 2019. Impact of selected antioxidant vitamins (Vitamin A, E and C) and micro minerals (Zn, Se) on the antioxidant status and performance under high environmental temperature in poultry. A review. Acta Agriculturae Scandinavica, Section A — Animal Science. DOI: 10.1080/09064702.2019.1611913

[57] Kucuk, O., N. Sahin, K. Sahin. 2003. Supplemental zinc and vitamin A can alleviate negative effects of heat stress in broiler chickens. Biological Trace Element Research. 3: 225-235.

[58] Mahmoud, K. Z., F.W. Edens. 2003. Influence of selenium sources on age-related and mild heat stress-related changes of blood and liver glutathione redox cycle in broiler chickens (Gallus domesticus). Comparative Biochemistry and Physiology Part B: Biochemistry and Molecular Biology. 4: 921-934.

[59] Mahmoud, K. Z., F.W. Edens, E.J. Eisen, G.B. Havenstein. 2004. Ascorbic acid decreases heat shock protein 70 and plasma corticosterone response in broilers (Gallus Domesticus) subjected to cyclic heat stress. Comparative Biochemistry and Physiology Part B: Biochemistry and Molecular Biology. 1: 35-42.

[60] Kumar, K., A. Mishra, A. A. Sheikh, P. Patel, M. K. Ahirwar, S. M. Bashir, A. Ali. 2017. Effect of Ascorbic Acid on

Some Biochemical Parameters during Heat Stress in Commercial Broilers. International Journal of Current Microbiology and Applied Sciences. 11: 5425-5434.

[61] Brandae-Neto, J.V., B.B. Stefan, W. Mendonca, A. Bloise, W.B. Castro 1995. The Essential Role Of Zinc In Growth. Nutritional Research. 15:.335–358.

[62] Nova, T.D., R. Zein. 2020. The optimization of ginger and Zinc in feed to preventing heat stress at tropical in local duck. IOP Conference Series: Earth and Environmental Science. 454. 012064. pp.1-9. DOI: 10.1088/ 1755-1315/454/1/012064.

[63] Roberson, K. D., H.M. Edwards Jr. 1994. Effects of 1, 25-dihydroxycholecalciferol and phytase on zinc utilization in broiler chicks. Poultry Science. 8: 1312-1326.

[64] Prasad, A. S., O. Kucuk. 2002. Zinc in cancer prevention. Cancer and Metastasis Reviews. 3-4: 291-295.

[65] Sahin, K., M. Onderci, N. Sahin, F. Gulcu, N. Yildiz, M. Avci, O. Kucuk. 2006. Responses of quail to dietary vitamin E and zinc picolinate at different environmental temperatures. Animal Feed Science and Technology. 1-2: 39-48.

[66] Kucuk, O. 2008. Zinc in a combination with magnesium helps reducing negative effects of heat stress in quails. Biological Trace Element Research. 1-3: 144-153.

[67] Suchý, P., E. Straková, I. Herzig. 2014. Selenium in poultry nutrition: a review. Czech Journal of Animal Science. 11: 495-503.

[68] Gallo-Torres, D.C. 1980. Absorption, blood transport, and metabolism of vitamin E. In: Machlin L. J. (Editor). A Comprehensive Treatise. New York: Marcel Dekker. 170–267.

[69] Park, J. H., S.N. Kang, D. Shin, K.S. Shim. 2015. Antioxidant enzyme activity and meat quality of meat type ducks fed with dried oregano (Origanumvulgare L.) powder. Asian-Australasian Journal of Animal Sciences. 1: 79-85.

[70] Samanya, M., K.E. Yamauchi. 2002. Histological alterations of intestinal villi in chickens fed dried Bacillus subtilis var. natto. Comparative Biochemistry and Physiology Part A: Molecular & Integrative Physiology. 1: 95-104.

[71] Hooge, D. M., H. Ishimaru, M.D. Sims. 2004. Influence of dietary Bacillus subtilis C-3102 spores on live performance of broiler chickens in four controlled pen trials. Journal of Applied Poultry Research. 2: 222-228.

[72] Li, W.F., I.R. Rajput, X. Xu, Y.L. Li, J. Lei, Q. Huang, M.Q. Wang. 2011. Effects of probiotic (Bacillus subtilis) on laying performance, blood biochemical properties and intestinal microflora of Shaoxing duck. International Journal of Poultry Science. 8: 583-589.

[73] Rajput, I. R., W.F. Li, Y.L. Li, L. Jian, M.Q. Wang. 2013.Application of probiotic (Bacillus subtilis) to enhance immunity, antioxidation, digestive enzymes activity and hematological profile of Shaoxing duck. Pakistan Veterinary Journal. 1: 69-72.

[74] Rahman, C. Hidayat. 2020. Reducing negative effect of heat stress in broiler through nutritional and feeding strategy. IOP Conf. Ser.: *Earth Environ. Sci. Improving Tropical Animal Production for Food Security22-24 November 2019, South East Sulawesi,* Indonesia. 465:012034. DOI: 10.1088/ 1755-1315/465/1/012034

[75] Khatlab, A., A. Vesco, E. Goes, A. Neto, M. Menck-Soares, E. Gasparino. 2018. Short communication: Gender and heat stress effects on hypothalamic gene expression and feed intake in broilers.

Spanish Journal of Agricultural Research. 16:e04SC02. DOI: 10.5424/sjar/2018161-11737

[76] Del Vesco, A. P., A. S. Khatlab, E. S. R. Goes, K. S. Utsunomiya, J. S. Vieira, A. R. Oliveira Neto, E. Gasparino. 2017. Age related oxidative stress and antioxidant capacity in heat-stressed broilers. Animal. 11:1783–1790. DOI: 10.1017/S1751731117000386

[77] Quinteiro-Filho, W. M., A. V. S. Gomes, M. L. Pinheiro, A. Ribeiro, V. Ferraz-de-Paula, C. S. Astolfi-Ferreira, A. J. P. Ferreira, J. Palermo-Neto. 2012. Heat stress impairs performance and induces intestinal inflammation in broiler chickens infected with Salmonella Enteritidis. Avian Patholology. 41:421–427. DOI: 10.1080/03079457.2012.709315

[78] Attia, Y. A., M. A. Al-Harthi, A. S. El-Shafey, Y. A. Rehab, W. K. Kim. 2017. Enhancing tolerance of broiler chickens to heat stress by supplementation with vitamin E, vitamin C and/or probiotics. Annals Animal Science. 17(4): 1155–1169. DOI: https://doi.org/10.1515/aoas-2017-0012

[79] Imik, H., M. A. Atasever, S. Urcar, H. Ozlu, R. Gumus, M. Atasever. 2012. Meat quality of heat stress exposed broilers and effect of protein and vitamin E. British Poultry Science. 53: 689–698. DOI: 10.1080/00071668.2012.736609

[80] Quinteiro-Filho, W. M., A. Ribeiro, V. Ferraz-de-Paula, M. L. Pinheiro, M. Sakai, L. R. S_a, A. J. Ferreira, J. Palermo-Neto. 2010. Heat stress impairs performance parameters, induces intestinal injury, and decreases macrophage activity in broiler chickens. Poultry Science. 89:1905–1914. DOI: 10.3382/ps.2010-00812

[81] Alhenaky, A., A. Abdelqader, M. Abuajamieh, A. R. Al Fataftah. 2017. The effect of heat stress on intestinal integrity and Salmonella invasion in broiler birds. Journal of Thermal Biology. 70:9–14. DOI: 10.1016/j.jtherbio.2017.10.015

[82] Marchini, C., E. Fernandes, M. Nascimento, E. Araújo, E. Guimarães, J. Bueno, N. Fagundes, M. Café. 2018. The effect of cyclic heat stress applied to different broiler chicken brooding stages on animal performance and carcass yield. Brazilian Journal of Poultry Science. 20:765–772. DOI: 10.1590/1806-9061-2017-0672

[83] Awad, E., M. Najaa, Z. Zulaikha, I. Zulkifli, A. Soleimani. 2020. Effects of heat stress on growth performance, selected physiological and immunological parameters, caecal microflora, and meat quality in two broiler strains. Asian-Australasian Journal of Animal Sciences. 33(5): 778–787. DOI: 10.5713/ajas.19.0208

[84] Attia, Y. A., S.S. Hassan. 2017. Broiler tolerance to heat stress at various dietary protein/energy levels. European Poultry Science. 81. DOI: 10.1399/eps.2017.171

[85] Al-Sultan, S. I., S. M. Abdel-Raheem, S. M. S. Abd-Allah, A. M. Edris. 2019. Alleviation of chronic heat stress in broilers by dietary supplementation of novel feed additive combinations. Slovenian Veterinary Research, 56 (Suppl. 22): 269–279.

[86] Ding, J., S. He, Y. Xiong, D. Liu, S. Dai, H. Hu. 2020. Effects of dietary supplementation of fumaric acid on growth performance, blood hematological and biochemical profile of broiler chickens exposed to chronic heat stress. Brazilian Journal of Poultry Science. 22 (01). DOI: 10.1590/1806-9061-2019-1147

[87] Sohail, M. U., M. E. Hume, J. A. Byrd, D. J. Nisbet, A. Ijaz, A. Sohail, M. Z. Shabbir, H. Rehman. 2012. Effect of supplementation of prebiotic mannan-

oligosaccharides and probiotic mixture on growth performance of broilers subjected to chronic heat stress. Poultry Science. 91:2235–2240. DOI: 10.3382/ps.2012-02182

[88] Jahromi, M. F., Y. W. Altaher, P. Shokryazdan, R. Ebrahimi, M. Ebrahimi, Z. Idrus, V. Tufarelli, J. B. Liang. 2016. Dietary supplementation of a mixture of lactobacillus strains enhances performance of broiler chickens raised under heat stress conditions. International Journal of Biometeorology. 60:1099-1110. DOI: 10.1007/s00484-015-1103-x

[89] Olfati, A, A. Mojtahedin, T. Sadeghi, M. Akbari, F. Martínez-Pastor. 2018. Comparison of growth performance and immune responses of broiler chicks reared under heat stress, cold stress and thermoneutral conditions. Spanish Journal of Agricultural Research. 16(2): e0505. DOI:10.5424/sjar/2018162-12753

[90] Ma, B., X. He, Z. Lu, L. Zhang, J. Li, Y. Jiang, G. Zhou, F. Gao. 2018. Chronic heat stress affects muscle hypertrophy, muscle protein synthesis and uptake of amino acid in broilers via insulin like growth factor-mammalian target of rapamycin signal pathway. Poultry Science. 97:4150–4158. DOI: 10.3382/ps/pey291

[91] Goo, D., J. H. Kim, G. Park, J. Reyes, D. Kil. 2019. Effect of heat stress and stocking density on growth performance, Breast meat quality, and intestinal barrier function in broiler chickens. Animals. 9(3):107. DOI: 10.3390/ani9030107

[92] Goel, A. 2021. Heat stress management in poultry. Journal of Animal Physiology and Animal Nutrition. 00:1–10. DOI: 10.1111/jpn.13496

[93] Ortega, A. D. S. V., C. Szabó. 2021. Adverse effects of heat stress on the intestinal integrity and function of pigs and the mitigation capacity of dietary antioxidants: a review. Animals. 11(4): 1135. DOI: 10.3390/ani11041135

Chapter 6

Use of Aromatic Seeds as Feed Additives to Improve the Production of Anatolian Water Buffaloes

Taşkın Değirmencioğlu

Abstract

Buffaloes have a strong population of rumen microorganisms that can utilize different feeds. Other features that make this animal unique are its compatibility with nature, its ability to withstand difficulties, and the nutrient richness of animal products. Today, the emergence of residues such as animal origin diseases, pesticides and antibiotics in animal food products has led organic products to be preferred more by consumers. Due to the increase in consumption demand of natural products, the share of buffalo products in the world market is gradually increasing. Focusing on the use of natural additives in buffalo feeding is important for the diversity of healthy products. Examples of natural additives are cumin and fenugreek seeds. In addition to being natural products, these seeds are reported to have versatile functions in the animal body. The purpose of this chapter is to show how to use aromatic seeds as feed additives in the feeding of Anatolian water buffaloes. The chapter also includes various articles on the use of aromatic seeds in buffalo rations in international fields. This review focuses on the current research relating to the use of aromatic seeds as feed additives to improve the production of Anatolian water buffaloes. Based on the scientific results presented in this chapter, authors drew the following main conclusions: (1) The use of aromatic seeds as feed additives of Anatolian water buffaloes feeding enabled in enhancing milk production, without changing the taste and chemical composition of the milk. (2) Milk production can be improved up to 0.67 kg and 0.85 kg day-1 by adding 50 g Fenugreek seeds and 30 g Cumin seeds to the ration of buffaloes in the early lactation period. (3) The use of aromatic seeds in the feeding of water buffaloes has been proven therefore, their use in the buffalo sector should be encouraged.

Keywords: Cumin seeds, fenugreek seeds, feed consumption, milk yield, organic animal

1. Introduction

With the increase in population, the product range for commercial purposes has gradually expanded in the food industry. Especially in the feed sector, new feed sources, corn chips, biscuits and chocolate residues were offered to animals. However, the reliability of these feed sources is a matter of debate. In intensive dairy buffaloes, green feeds are harvested and brought to the feet of the animal. Buffalo cows are fed with blended feed consisting of alfalfa hay, corn silage, straw, concentrate feed and sometimes food agricultural residues (such as tomato peel, beer grinder residues, sugar beet pulp). The Anatolian buffalo has a great potential in terms of organic animal husbandry because of its resistance to diseases, its diet based on pasture, not adding synthetic additives to its feed, and its usefulness for human health. On the other hand, considering the insufficient technological and economic infrastructure of the breeders, the drying of wetlands to agriculture, the risk of drug residues, the use of genetically modified feed in feed factories, the above-mentioned negative effects constitute a serious risk in terms of this potential [1]. Organic (ecological, biological) animal production is a production method of ecological balance, animal welfare and product quantity, criteria of health criteria in product quality [2]. In organic animal production enterprises, species and breeds which are resistant to environmental and climatic conditions and diseases should be selected [3]. Buffaloes are resistant to sudden feed changes and can feed on low-quality forages. They are also resistant to diseases caused by blood parasites in their feet and mouth, namely BSE, IBR-IPV [4]. Therefore, because the Anatolian water buffalo does not need a special care, they are sought for organic livestock. In organic livestock, hormones, antibiotics and the like substances cannot be used to speed up the growth rate and maximize the feed utilization. Genetically modified (GMO) feeds, chemically treated feeds or synthetic additives cannot be used [5]. Studies have been carried out to improve natural consumption and rumen conditions as well as natural additives in rations of Anatolian water buffaloes. As example of this additive can be given aromatic plants [6]. As it is known, the milk yield of an animal after giving birth reaches its peak level in 8–10 weeks. On the contrary, the ability to consume food can not rise rapidly to meet the increase in milk yield [7]. The energy imbalance seen in this period is called as negative energy balance [8]. During this period, animals try to compensate their energy insufficiency by breaking up fat tissues in their bodies. The risk of metabolic disease increases significantly when fat breakdown exceeds physiological limits [9]. In this period, however, the use of aromatic plants in livestock increases feed consumption, thereby reducing the energy imbalance The milk yield-increasing effect of aromatic seeds has been investigated mainly in ruminants. The milk productivity of AWB is very low because of traditionally feeding based on pasture. Milk supply can be increase with some herbal in cattle.

2. Anatolian water Buffalo

Buffaloes in our country have their origins in the Mediterranean buffalo, one of the subspecies of river buffaloes, and are defined as the Anatolian water buffalo (AWB). (Bubalusbubalis). It is a domestic race registered by the race registration committee with the communiqué dated 12.12.2004 and numbered 25668 of the Official Gazette 2004/39 [10]. The AWB showing a distribution to all parts of Turkey mainly the Black Sea region and the north of the Central Anatolia has a live weight ranging between 400 and 450 kg in adult females and 450–500 kg in adult males. It has a height of 129 to 136 cm in the shoulder region (cidago height). The AWB has a rough, angular and muscular body, a low rump and thick and strong joints. The hair color is black and dark gray in adult buffaloes. Some individuals may have whiteness at their heads, feet and tails (**Figure 1**).

The lactation period ranges between 200 and 250 days and the total milk yield in the lactation period ranges between 800 and 1000 kg. The fat ratio in the milk varies between 6 and 8% [11]. During the Ottoman Empire period, Turks passing to the Balkans took their buffaloes with them. The Turkish buffalo spread to a wide area

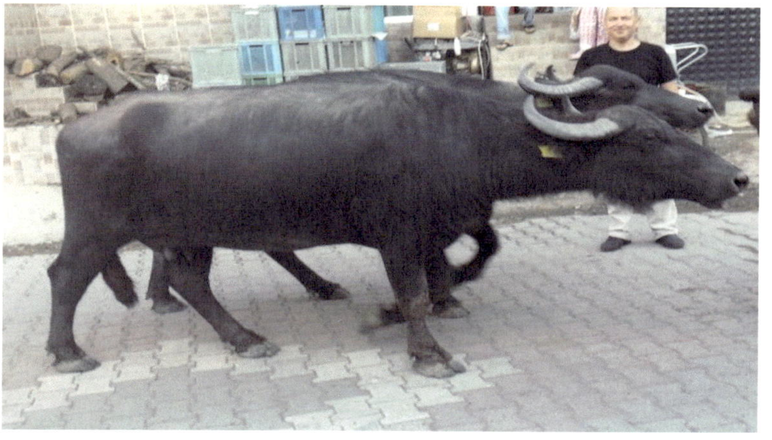

Figure 1.
Anatolian water Buffalo (Bupalusbupalis).

in the Balkan countries with wet and fertile lands (Mecadonia, Western Thrace and Bulgaria) [1]. There is a wide range of AWB products. For example, Ney is the only woodwind of Turkish Classical Music and the head instrument of Turkish Sufi Music. Ney is one of the instruments whose sound is closest to human voice. A mouthpiece called baspare is attached on the top hole in order to obtain a clearer sound and to prevent the lips from being hurt. Baspare is usually made of water buffalo horn. Similarly, buffalo horn is used in the production of Turkish bows and combs. Yoghurt, cream and mozzarella cheese are made from its milk and sausages are made from its meat. According to the recent scientific findings it can be stated that milk and meat yields of buffaloes are lower than those of cattle. However, products obtained from buffalo can be sold at a low cost and a higher price than cattle [12].

3. Aromatic seeds

The Saponins are naturally occurring surface-active glycosides. Chemically, saponins are high-molecular-weight glycosides in which sugars (glycone) (1–8 residues) are linked to a triterpene or steroidal aglyconemoiety [13]. Johnson et al. [14] found that some saponins increase the permeability of intestinal mucosal cells. Herbal containing saponin can contribute to nutrient requirements, stimulate the endocrine system and affect intermediate nutrient metabolism [15, 16]. In addition saponin-rich materials increase the partitioning of nutrients towards microbial mass, mainly by affecting protein degradation and by having anti-protozoal effects [17]. The seeds of fenugreek and cumin contain alkaloids, flavonoids, saponins, amino acids, tannins and some steroidal glycosides [18].

Fenugreek seeds (FS) (*Trigonellafoenumgraecum*) is an annual crop belonging to the legume family [19]. Fenugreek has a positive effect on the lactation performance of ruminants. Diocin is a natural saponin found in Fenugreek and has a structural similarity to estrogen [20].

There are two main purposes of grinding the fenugreek substance. The first is to separate the grain into small particles that can be found in the same proportion throughout the mixed feed. The other should be given roughly broken in order to facilitate digestion in buffaloes. Otherwise, a significant portion of the seeds is thrown out without being digested. Treatment of grinding fenugreek seeds proceeded at 3-mm intervals (**Figure 2**).

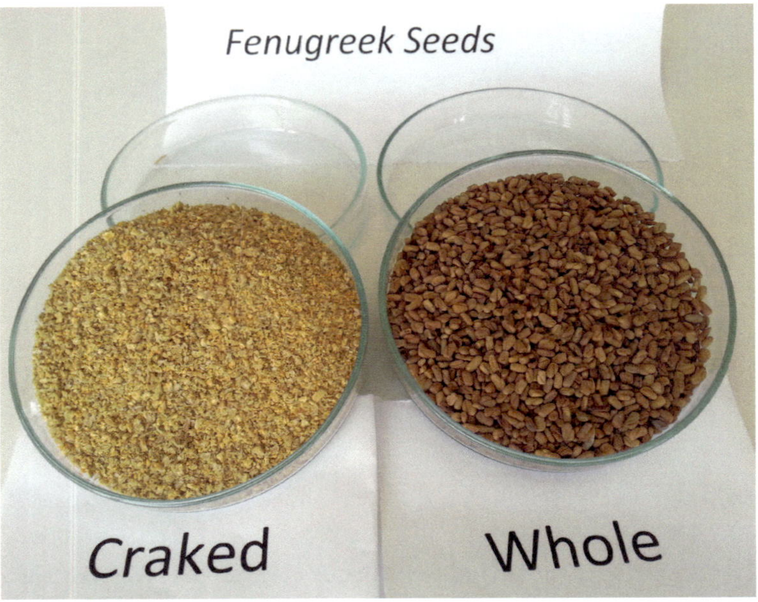

Figure 2.
The form of the fenugreek seed used in trial.

Cumin seeds (CS), whose scientific name is *Cuminumcyminum* L. and belonging to the apiacea family is a well-known herbal medicine in Iran [21]. Its fruits contain 2–5% volatile oil, usually obtained by steam distillation of the dried and crushed fruits. This oil has the ability to easily diffuse across cell membrane to induce biological reactions. Cuminaldehyde is one of the major flavoring components of cumin essential oil that can induce different biological activities. Previous studies showed that the antimicrobial and fungitoxic activity could be linked to the main compound, cuminic aldehyde [22]. Positive effects of CS on feed consumption in ruminants have been reported by some researchers [23, 24].

This herbal is a very good source of iron which is a mineral that plays many vital roles in the body. CS has traditionally been noted to be of benefit for digestive system and also has anti-carcinogenic properties [25]. Moreover, Cumin fruit has been used to stimulate breast milk production in Iranian traditional medicine [26]. The nutrient composition of seed depending on the raw material source and the storage conditions. Many studies have shown that the protein content of FS varies between 27.42–42%, and However, the oil content was low, below 10%, Linolenic acid (18: 3) was present at low relative level (below 1.0%) [27], totalcarbohydrate 56.14%, neutral detergent fiber 18.62%, acid detergent fiber % 4.38 and hemi cellulose 14.24% [28]. The chemical composition of FS and CS respectively contained on dry matter basis (DM) 91.11 and 92.43%, crude protein (CP) 29.49 and 19.64%, ether extract (EE) 3.86 and 15.68%, crude ash (CA) 3.23 and 6.95% ME 2373.67 and 2461.07 kcal/kg. Chemicalcomposition of FS and CS seeds are presented in **Table 1**.

As can be seen in **Table 1**, crude cellulose content of FCS and CS and was 6.20 and 11.23% depending on the crust ratio in the seed. The chemical composition of FS and CS respectively contained on dry matter basis (DM) 91.11 and 92.43%, crude protein (CP) 29.49 and 19.64%, ether extract (EE) 3.86 and 15.68%, crude ash (CA) 3.23 and 6.95% ME 2373.67 and 2461.07 kcal/kg (**Table 1**).

The crude protein of FS is higher than the CS. However, the ether extract, cellulose, crude ash, ADF and NDF content of the CS was higher compared with the FS.

Feed	DM	OM	CP	EE	CE	CA	NFE	ADF	NDF	ME (kcal kg^{-1})
Fen.	91.11	87.88	29.49	3.86	6.20	3.23	48.33	11.50	14.44	2373.67
Cum.	92,43	85.48	19.64	15.68	11.23	6.95	38.93	20.66	44.90	2461.07

Cumin DM: Dry Matter; OM: Organic Matter; CP: Crude Protein; EE: Ether Extract; CE: Cellulose; CA: Crude Ash; NFE: Nitrogen Free Extract; ADF: Acid Detergent-Fiber; NDF: Neutral Detergent Fiber; ADL: Acid Detergent Lignin; ME: Metabolizable Energy calculated according to the equation of [29].

Table 1.
Chemical composition of fenugreek [30] and cumin seeds [31] DM (%).

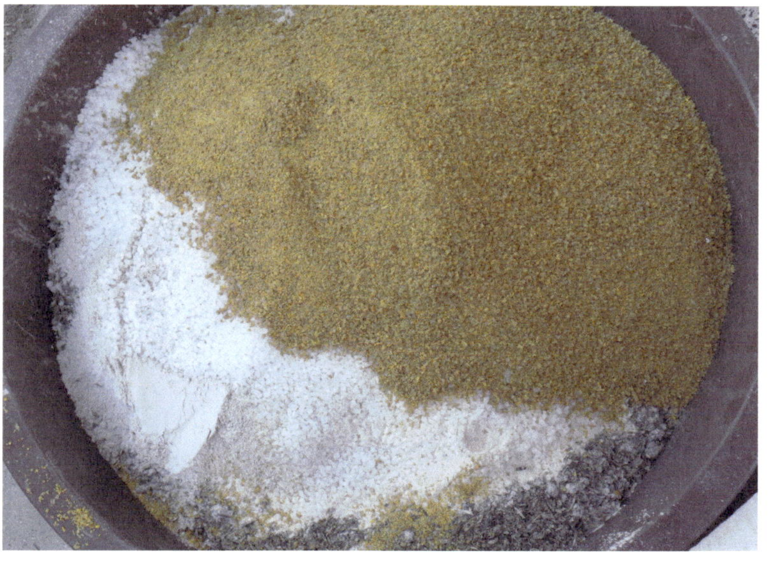

Figure 3.
Concentrate feed mixture (CFM).

In addition to the crude protein content of over 29%, fenugreek seeds are increasingly replacing plant-based meal feeds with its nutrient profile.

Experimental rations were as follows: control Concentrate feed mixture-(CFM) and CFM consisted of 31% barley, 32% wheat, 30% sunflower meal, treated 5% Fenugreek seed 1% marble powder, 0.75% salt and 0.25% vitamin+ mineral mix (**Figure 3**) [30].

3.1 The use of aromatic seeds in buffaloes

To summarize thousands of studies on aromatic seeds in this review it does not seem possible. Therefore, this chapter focuses only on the most important aromatic seeds those can be considered in buffaloes feeding.

3.2 The effects of aromatic seeds on dry matter intake

Daily intake of dry matter (DM) in an animal defines its capability of feed consumption. Dry matter consumption; It is affected by factors such as animal factor, environmental factor and feed [1]. Positive effects of aromatic seeds on dry matter intake in buffaloes have been reported by some researchers. When studies on milk buffaloes were examined, it was seen that aromatic seeds were used in early lactation buffalo rations.

Değirmencioglu et al. [30] 24 lactating Anatolian buffaloes at lactation stage 30–45 days of lactation were randomly selected and distributed into two different groups with 12animals in each group. Animals in Group I fed by control ration and in Group II fed by control ration plus fenugreek seeds (GFS) 50 g kg^{-1}. In a related study, Total DM consumption in group 2 was higher than in the control group 1 (5.92% (P < 0:05)); it was determined that the grinding fenugreek seeds (GFS) at a level of 5% had a significant effect on dry matter consumption (0.83 kg/day) in buffalo rations (**Table 2**) [30].

In another study, Değirmencioğlu et al. [31] A total of 27 multifarious AWB at stage 40–50 days of lactation were randomly selected and distributed into three different groups with 9 animals in each group. Animals in Group I fed by control ration, in Group II fed by control ration plus cumin seeds (GCS) 10 g kg^{-1} and in Group III fed by control ration plus 30 g GCS kg^{-1}. GCS application significantly increasedto a total DM consumption (P < 0.01; 11.69,12.14 and 13.01 kg day^{-1} for S1, S2 and S3 diets, respectively). The total DM consumption washigher in buffaloes fed by S3 diet than in buffaloesfed by the S2 and S1 diets (6.68% and 10.14%, P < 0.01) (**Table 3**) [31].

Parameter	**Groups**		**Significance**
	Group I (Control) n = 12	**5% (GFS)[1] Group II n = 12**	
Total DM intake[2]	13.17 ± 0.41	14.00 ± 0.34	*
Milkyield (kg d^{-1})	7.34 ± 0.24	8.01 ± 0.19	**
Fat (%)	5.80 ± 0.19	6.06 ± 0.17	NS
SNF (%)	10.18 ± 0.05	10.30 ± 0.04	NS
Protein (%)	4.95 ± 0.15	5.11 ± 0.21	NS
SCC(x log10 mL^{-1})	60.35 ± 6.83	53.70 ± 7.57	NS

[1]*Ground fenugreek seed (GFS).*
[2]*Total DM intake values for buffaloes were not added to pasture consumption. 4% FCM = 4% fat-corrected milk; SNF=Solids-not-fat; SCC = Somatic Cell Count; SE = Standard error, NS = Not significant; The difference between the treatment was significant at P = 5% (*) and 1% (**) level, respectively.*

Table 2.
The effects of grounding fenugreek seeds on the performance of Anatolian water buffalo (mean ± SE) [30].

Parameter	**Groups**			**Significance 2**
	Group I (Control) n = 9	**1% (GCS)[1] Group II n = 9**	**Group III 3% GCS n = 9**	
Total DM intake[2]	11.69 ± 0.20[a]	12.14 ± 0.20[a]	13.01 ± 0.27[b]	**
Milkyield (kg d^{-1})	5.83 ± 0.09[a]	6.17 ± 0.14[a]	6.68 ± 1.28[b]	**
4% FCM	7.73 ± 0.21[a]	7.46 ± 0.25[ab]	8.38 ± 0.19[b]	*
Fat (%)	6.27 ± 0.32	5.45 ± 0.30	5.62 ± 0.25	NS
SNF (%)	10.32 ± 0.08	10.14 ± 0.06	10.15 ± 0.06	NS
Protein (%)	4.53 ± 0.10	4.24 ± 0.08	4.20 ± 0.07	NS
SCC(x log10 mL^{-1})	159.74 ± 39.00	153.78 ± 20.51	92.29 ± 9.60	NS

[1]*Ground cumin seed (GCS) SE = Standard error, NS = Not significant; The difference between the treatment was significant at P = 5% (*) and 1% (**) level, respectively. Different superscripts in the same row indicate significant differences among treatments. Significant levels are defined in the footnote of* **Table 2.**

Table 3.
The effects of grounding cuminum seeds on the performance of Anatolian water buffalo (mean ± SE) [31].

In another study, Kirar et al. [32] 12 lactating Murrah buffaloes of 1st to3 parity were randomly selected and distributed into two different groups with six animals in each group. Animals in Group I were control without any supplementation and in Group II were supplemented with soaked fenugreek seeds 50 g per animal per day (**Table 4**) [32].

In another study, Choubey et al. [28] a total of 18 lactating Surti buffalos at stage 55.52 ± 8.61 day of lactation) were selected and divided into 3 homogenous groups with 6 animals in each group. Animals in Group I fed by control ration, in Group II fed by control ration plus fenugreek seeds (GFS) 1.5% and in Group III fed by control ration plus 3.0% FS. During the research, organaleptic taste tastes were determined in the milk obtained from I, II and III groups. 6.47, 6.80 and 6.84 As a result of the study, it was determined that the use of fenugreek in milk did not affect the aromatic structure of the milk negatively (**Table 5**) [28].

As it can be seen in **Tables 2** and **3**, it is seen that the use of aromatic seeds in the ration has a significant effect on the total dry matter intake of buffaloes.

Parameters	Group I Control diet n = 6	Group II 50 g FS[1]/head n = 6
Milkyield (kg d^{-1})	5.40 ± 0.13	6.80 ± 0.08
Fat (%)	6.47 ± 0.11	6.45 ± 0.11
Milk SNF (%)	9.63 ± 0.10	9.95 ± 0.15
Milk protein (%)	3.57 ± 0.05	3.55 ± 0.06
Milk lactose (%)	4.95 ± 0.08	5.08 ± 0.06

[1]*Fenugreek seed (FS).*

Table 4.
Effect of fenugreek on the performance of Murrah buffaloes (mean ± SE) [32].

Parameter	Groups			Significance[2]
	Group I (Control) n = 6	Group II 1.5% FS[1] n = 6	Group III 3.0% FS n = 6	
Milkyield (kg d^{-1})	3.72^a ± 0.20	4.05^b ± 0.22	3.87^{ab} ± 0.34	0.049
Fat (%)	8.21 ± 0.86	8.19 ± 0.86	7.72 ± 0.77	0.697
Density	31.94 ± 1.40	32.99 ± 0.88	33.01 ± 0.51	0.452
SNF (%)	9.95 ± 0.37	10.24 ± 0.13	10.10 ± 0.20	0.453
Protein (%)	4.19 ± 0.21	4.33 ± 0.16	4.44 ± 0.25	0.442
Laktose (%)	5.10 ± 0.17	5.15 ± 0.18	5.15 ± 0.07	0.806
Appearance	6.47 ± 0.09	7.06 ± 0.08	7.24 ± 0.09	0.133
Flavor	6.51 ± 0.09	6.76 ± 0.05	6.80 ± 0.13	0.060
Palatability	6.47 ± 0.11	6.80 ± 0.11	6.84 ± 0.16	0.073

[1]*Fenugreek seed (FS).*
[2]*Different superscripts in the same row indicate significant differences among treatments. Significant levels are defined in the footnote of* **Table 2**.

Table 5.
Effect of fenugreek on the performance of Surti buffaloes (mean ± SE) [28].

The positive effects on DM consumption of aromatic seeds could be explained by effect hypothalamus to stimulate hunger centers in the brain and increasing the desire for eating [33]. Fenugreek may also increase food consumption through inhibition of leptin secretion [34]. In addition, due to the rich nutrient content of aromatic seeds, increases the number of rumen microorganisms, which positively affects the degradability of roughage.

3.3 The effects on milk production

As it can be seen in **Tables 2-5**, in the case of using aromatic seeds in the water buffalo's diet, this could be resulted in significant increasing in milk yield 8.36%, 12.72%, ($P < 0:01$) 20.58%($P > 0:01$) and 8.14%.

Fenugreek seeds contain a fair amount of steroidal saponnin which may improve the nutrient absorption by altering the mucosal permeability of intestine [35]. Stimulation of endogenous hormone secretion could be hypothesized through a mechanism by which fenugreek exerts its action on milk yield. In buffaloes, fenugreek feeding increased plasma levels of prolactin [36]. However, the role of this hormone in the lactating ruminants is not far away from understanding [37, 38]. Present results indicate that growth hormone might be a possible candidate as a mediator of fenugreek action on milk production. Growth hormone (GH) is known to have a strong galactopoietic effect on lactation performance in ruminants since the exogenous administration of bovine somatotropin stimulates milk yield [39]. GH levels reported to increase in response to fenugreek feeding [40]. These seeds posses, an estrogen like substance which is also supposed to accomplish its galactagogue role [41–43] observed that the herbs increased in milk production by stimulating the endogenous hormonal secretion in mammals. They have also proved their worth as component of herbal preparation to improve the lactation performance and health of dairy buffalo [30] found an improvement in milk yield (0.67 kg/day) through supplementation of grounded FS (50 g/kg in concentrate) in Anatolian water buffaloes (**Table 2**). Other researchers [28, 32], like showed that supplementation of fenugreek seeds (100 g/day) and (% 1.5) on lactating Murrah buffaloes and surti buffaloes resulted in a increase in milk production although nonsignificant, no change in milk composition (**Tables 4** and 5). With the progress of experiment, there appeared an improvement in the daily milk yield due to supplementation of soaked fenugreek seeds at both the dosage level. It was decided to be used of lowest dosage in diet so that could not pass bad smell into milk and as well as economic costing [30]. Değirmencioğlu et al. [31] also reported that supplementation of 30 g cumin seeds significantly ($P < 0.01$) increased mean daily milk production (0.85 kg) in Anatolian water buffaloes (**Table 3**). In these studies, CS and FS supplementation did not affect milk composition of buffalo and this result complies with the other studies [28, 32] who reported that differences in SNF, protein and fat contents of buffalo milk fed ration supplemented with SC were not significant (**Tables 4** and 5). Conversely, [25] showed that milk protein contents were significantly ($P < 0.05$) affected by CS supplementation. Similarly [44] reported that decreasing in milk fat of goats due to FS supplementation at very high dosage. There was a concern that the pungent aroma or taste of the fenugreek seeds could be transmitted to milk and alter milk flavor. Some of the prior studies, suspect that a higher dose supplementation of any herbal supplement having distinct aroma or taste may impart off flavor to milk [45]. Each raw milk sample was tasted to assess sweetness, saltiness, bitterness or rancidity. Thus a sensory evaluation was carried out to determine the organoleptic acceptability of milk. Shah and Mir [46] reported that dietary fenugreek seeds did not adversely affect milk production, DM intake and organoleptic acceptability of milk of cows, and can be used to improve milk quality by reducing milk cholesterol content and increasing desirable functional fatty acids in milk. Similarly researcher determined a positive effect on the flavor and palatability of milk with increasing fenugred dose p = 0.060 and p = 0.073 (**Table 5**) [28]. This can be explained by the powerful antioxidant effect of fenugreek. It is stated that the milk with fenugreek prevents oxidative loss in the fat during heating, and thus a flavor and aromatic structure is formed in the milk [47].

4. Conclusion

Based on the scientific results presented in this chapter, the following main conclusions can be drawn:

1. The use of aromatic seeds as feed additives of Anatolian water buffaloes feeding enabled in enhancing milk production, without changing the taste and chemical composition of the milk.

2. Milk production can be improved upto 0.67 kg and 0.85 kg day^{-1} by adding 50 g Fenugreek seeds and 30 g Cumin seeds to the ration of buffaloes in the early lactation period.

3. The use of aromatic seeds in the feeding of water buffaloes has been proven therefore, their use in the buffalo sector should be encouraged.

Author details

Taşkın Değirmencioğlu
Department of Milk and Fattening, Karacabey Vocational School, Bursa Uludag University, Bursa, Republic of Turkey

*Address all correspondence to: taskin@uludag.edu.tr

References

[1] Değirmencioğlu, T[a]. 2020 The Nutrition of Buffaloes," ISBN: 978-625-402-317-0. Nobel publishing house. Ankara. 320 p

[2] Y. Sayan, and M. Polat, "Ekolojik Tarımda Hayvancılık". Türkiye 2.Ek. Tar. Semp. 14-16 Antalya. 2001, pp 95-104.

[3] Anonim, "Organik Tarımın Esaslarıve Uygulamasınaİlişkin Yönetmelik" http://www.resmigazete.basbakanlik.gov.tr/eskiler/2010/08/20100818. htm. 2010.

[4] Anonymous, "T.C. Tarımveköyişlerib akanlığıtarımsalaraştırmagenelmüdürl üğü," Türkiyeevcilhayvangenetikkaynakl arıtanıtımkataloğu, 22s. http://www.tarim.gov.tr/TAGEM/Belgeler/yayin/Katalog%20Türkçe.pdf. 2009.

[5] Anonim,"Organik Tarımın EsaslarıveUygulamasınaİlişkin Yönetmelik" http://www.resmigazete.basbakanlik.gov.tr/eskiler/2010/08/20100818. htm. 2010.

[6] Değirmencioğlu, T. 2018. 'Anatolian Water Buffalo's Role in the Organic Animal Product' 11th International Conference on Agriculture, Biological, Environmental and Medical Sciences (ABEMS-18), Bangkok (Thailant) 51-56.

[7] Bell A.W., 1995. "Regulation of organic nutrient metabolism during transition from late pregnancy to early lactation". J. Anim.Sci., 73:2804-2819.

[8] Gorgulu, M. 2009. "Büyükve Küçükbaş Hayvan Besleme", Çukurova Üniv. ZiraatFak., Ders Notu, 282 s.

[9] Knaus, W.F. Steinwidder, A.and W. Zolltsc, 2001 "Energy and Protein Balance in Organic Dairy Cow Nutrition-Model Calculations Based on EU Regulations In: Breeding and Feeding For Animal Helath and Welfare in Organic Livestock Systems", Proceedings of the Fourth NAHWOA Workshop, 24-27 March, Wageningen, Holland

[10] Anonymous, http://www.mevzuat.gov.tr/Metin.Aspx?MevzuatKod=9.5.6109&MevzuatIliski=0&sourceXmlSearch. 2016.

[11] Atasever, S and Erdem, H "Manda YetiştiriciliğiveTürkiye'dekiGeleceği". O.M.Ü. Zir. Fak.Derg., 23(1):59-64. 2008.

[12] Kucukkebabcı, M and Aslan S. 2002, "Evcildişimandalardaüremeözellik". Lala.,HayvAraştEnstDerg, 42 (2): 55-63.

[13] Hostettmann, K., and Marston, A.: Saponins. Cambridge: Cambridge University Press, 1995.

[14] Johnson IT, Gee JM, Price K, Curl C, Fenwick GR, 1986. Influence of saponins on gut permeability and active nutrient transport in vitro. J. Nutri., 116: 2270-2277.

[15] Wang Y, McAllister TA, Yanke LJ, Cheeke PR, et al. 2000. Effect of steroidal saponin from Yucca schidigeraextract on ruminal microbes. J. App. Microbiol. 88: 887-896.

[16] Wenk C. 2000. Why all discussion about herbs?. Biotechn. In the feed industry. proc. of alltech's 16th Annu. Symp. Alltech technical publications, Nottginham Univ. Press. Nicholasvile, KY.79-96.

[17] Goel, G., Makkar, P.S.H., and Becker, K.: Effects of Sesbaniasesban and Carduuspycnocephalus leaves and Fenugreek (Trigonellafoenum-graecum L.) seeds and their extracts on partitioning of nutrients from roughage- and concentrate-based feeds to methane, Animal Feed Science and Technology, 147, 72-89. 2008.

[18] Yadav R., Tiwari R., 2011 Chowdhary P., and Pradhan C.K.: A pharmacognostical monograph of trigonellafoenum- graecum seeds, Int J Pharm PharmSci, Vol 3, Suppl 5, 442-445, 2011.

[19] Acharya, S., Srichamroen, A., Basu, S., Ooraikul, B., and Basu, T.: Improvement in the nutraceutical properties of fenugreek (Trigonellafoenum-graecum L.), Songklanakarin J. Sci. Technol. Vol.28 (Suppl.1), 2006.

[20] IndhuPrathibha A, BhanuRekha V, Ajay Kumar VJ, NithyaQuintoil M and Abhishek Madan 2020 The Pharma Innovation Journal Interventions in feeding systems and management of dairy animals- food security strategy in livestock sector 9(8): 109-111

[21] Tuncturk R, Tuncturk M. 2006. Effects of different phosphorus levels on the yield and quality components of cumin (Cuminumcyminum L.)Res.j. Agric.Biol. Sci.2:336-340.

[22] De M, De AK, Mukhopadhyay R, Banerjee AB, Miro M et al. 2003. Antimicrobial activity of Cuminumcyminum L. ArsPharmaceutica, 44(3): 257-269.

[23] Hammer KA, Carson CF, Riley TV. 1999 Antimicrobial activity of essential oils and other plant extracts. Journal of Applied Microbiology, 86, 985-990.

[24] Khan MMH, Chaudhry AS. 2010. Chemical composition of selected forages and spices and the effect of these spices on in vitro rumen degradability of some forages Asian-Aust. J. Anim. Sci., 23 p. 889-900.

[25] Nurdin E, Arief. 2009. The Effectivity of Cumin as natural-antioxidant to improve rumen ecology of mastitis dairy cow's. JurnalProduksiTernak (University of JenderalSoedirman). 11(3):114-119.

[26] Hashemian N, GhasemiPirbalouti A, Hashemi M, Golparvar A, Hamedi B, et al. 2013. Diversity in chemical composition and antibacterial activity of essential oils of cumin (Cuminumcyminum L.) diverse from northeast of Iran. Aust. J. Crop Sci. 7: 1752-1760.

[27] Nour Ahmed Osman, Salah Elhussein, Ahmed Abdurrahman Taha2015 Content of Crude Protein, Fixed Oil and Lecithin in Sudanese Seed Accessions of Fenugreek (Trigonellafoenum-graecum L.) Pakistan Journal of Nutrition 14(12):907-912 DOI: 10.3923/pjn.2015.907.912

[28] Choubey, M Patel, V R Raval A P and singh R R 2018 Effect of fenugreek seed supplementation on lactation performance of Surti buffaloes Indian Journal of Animal Sciences 88 (3): 322-325, March 2018/Article

[29] Lodhi, G.N., Singh, D., and Ichponani, J.S. 1976: Variation in nutrient content of feedstuffs rich in protein and reassessment of the chemical methods for metabolizable energy estimation for poultry. J. Agric. Sci. Camb., 86, 293-303.

[30] Değirmencioglu, T., UnaL, H., Ozbilgin, S. Kuraloglu, H. 2016. " Effect of Ground Fenugreek Seeds (Trigonellafoenumgraecum) on Feed Consumption and Milk Performance in Anatolian Water Buffaloes" Arch. Anim. Breed, Arch. Anim. Breed., 59 (3): 345-349. Germany Doi: 10.5194/aab-59-345-2016

[31] Değirmencioğlu,T[b]. Şimşek, E., Unal,H., Kuraloğlu,H., Özbilgin., S. 2020. 'Effect of cumin seeds (cuminumcyminum) in feed diets of anatolian water buffaloes on shelter into gass concentration, milk yield and composition" Bulletin of University of Agricultural Sciences and Veterinary Medicine Cluj-Napoca. Animal Science and Biotechnologies 77(1):41-50.

[32] Kirar, M. Ghosh, S.. Baghel , R.P.S. Jain, A. Lakhani G.P, Roy B. and Jain A.K 2018 Int. J. Curr. Microbiol. App. Sci 7(7): 70-77

[33] Petit, P., Sauvaire, Y., Ponsin, G., Manteghetti, M., Fave,A., and Ribes,G.: 1993 Effects of a fenugreek seed extract on fedingbehaviour in the rat: Metabolic endocrine correlates. Pharmacol. Biochem.Behav., 45, 369-374,

[34] Kandhare, A.D.; Bandyopadhyay, D.; Thakurdesai, P.A. Low molecular weight galactomannans-based standardized fenugreek seed extract ameliorates high-fat diet-induced obesity in mice via modulation of FASn, IL-6, leptin, and TRIP-Br2. RSC Adv. 2018, 8, 32401-32416. [CrossRef]

[35] Pandian R S, Anuradha C V and Viswanathan P. 2002. Gastroprotective effect of fenugreek seeds (Trigonellafoenumgraecum) on experimental gastric ulcer in rats. Journal of Ethnopharmacology 81: 393-97.

[36] Abo-EL-Nor, S.A.H., 1999. Influence of fenugreek seeds as a galactagogue on milk yield, milk composition and different blood biochemical of lactating buffaloes during midlactation. Egypt. J. Dairy Sci., 27: 231-238.

[37] Hart, I.C., 1973. Effect of 2-Bromo-Ergocryptine on milk yield and the level of prolactin and growth hormone in the blood of the goat at milking. J. Endocrinol., 57: 179-180.

[38] Forsyth, I.A. and P.D. Lee, 1993. Bromocriptine treatment of periparturient goats: Long suppression of prolactin and lack of effect on lactation. J. Dairy Res., 60: 307-317.

[39] Bauman, D.E., 1992. Bovine somatotropin: Review of an emerging animal technology. J. Dairy Sci., 75: 3432-3451.

[40] Alamer M A and Basiouni G F. 2005. Feeding effects of fenugreek seeds (Trigonellafoenum-graecum L.) on lactation performance, some plasma constituents and growth hormone level in goats. Pakistan Journal of Biological Sciences 8: 1553-56.

[41] Tiran D. 2003. The use of fenugreek for breast feeding women. Complementary Therapies in Nursing and Midwifery 9: 155– 56.

[42] Kumar, S Mehla, R.K. and Dang, A.K 2008 "Use of shatavari (Asparagus racemosus) as a galactopoietic and therapeutic herb – a review". Agric. Rev. 29, 132-138.

[43] Bhatt N, Singh M, Ali A. 2009. Effect of feeding herbal preparations on milk yield and rumen parameters in lactating crossbred cows. Int. J. Agric. Biol. 11, 721-726.

[44] Balgees A, Atta Elmnan N M, Jame S A, Rahmatalla E O, Amasiab A and Mahala G. 2013. Effect of fenugreek (Trigonellafoenumgraecum) seeds supplementation on feed intake,some metabolic hormones profile, milk yield and composition of nubian goats. Research Journal of Animal Sciences 7: 1-5.

[45] Randby A T, Selmer-Olsen I and Baevre L. 1999. Effect of ethanol in feed on milk flavor and chemical composition. Journal of Dairy Science 82: 420-28.

[46] M. A. Shah and P. S. Mir 2004 Effect of dietary fenugreek seed on dairy cow performance and milk characteristics. CANADIAN JOURNAL OF ANIMAL SCIENCE 725-729

[47] Wani S A and Kumar P. 2016. Fenugreek: A review on its nutraceutical properties and utilization in various food products. Journal of the Saudi Society of Agricultural Sciences.(In press).doi: doi.10.1016/j. jssas.2016.01.007

Chapter 7

Microbial Inoculation to High Moisture Plant By-Product Silage: A Review

Bhutikini D. Nkosi, Cyprial N. Ncobela, Ronald S. Thomas, Ingrid M.M. Malebana, Francuois Müller, Sergio Álvarez and Robin Meeske

Abstract

Use of microbial inoculants during silage making have drawn interest to silage producers including those who are feeding their livestock on silage produced from by-products (e.g. pulps). Many farmers in the developing countries rely on agro-industrial by-products to feed their livestock, which is limited by the high moisture content of the by-products. This review pertains to issues related to silage production from high moisture plant by-products (e.g. pulps or pomaces), challenges involved in the ensiling of these resources, the use of additives (e.g. microbial additives), and growth performance of the animals that are fed silage from these resources. This information will be helpful to better understand the key roles of silage production from these resources.

Keywords: additives, digestion, forages, inoculation, methane, pulps

1. Introduction

The increasing demand for sustainable animal production is driving animal nutritionists to explore strategies for using high moisture by-products in animal feeding. Several researchers [1, 2] have reviewed the use of agro-industrial by-products as animal feed resources. These by-products are available during food processing and or beverage production, and are often produced in abundance, making it difficult to use them in a short period. Using these by-products in animal feeds will assist the food producing factories to reduce disposal costs while minimising the environmental impacts that these by-products would otherwise create [3].

The high moisture (>25%) content of these by-products makes it difficult to transport and handling during processing and storing [4]. While disposing these by-products might seem as a solution, such an act is associated with potential environmental pollution [5]. Subsequently, the high moisture coupled with high sugar content of these by-products allows for easy contamination by foreign materials and unwanted microbes, which leads to spoilage [1]. Despite the negative factors that are linked with these by-products, they contain valuable nutritional properties such as crude protein, organic matter, fibre and oil [1]. These resources should be processed and stored for animal feeding.

IntechOpen

The drying of high moisture by-products to produce meals for animal feeding is technically feasible, but is costly and laborious [6]. Research has shown that ensiling can be an alternative for processing and storing of these resources, provided all basic principles of ensiling are followed [7, 8]. Ensiling entails the preservation of plant/crop resources through anaerobic fermentation, usually by epiphytic bacteria that converts soluble carbohydrates to mainly lactic acid, and minor amounts of volatile fatty acids. The production of organic acids during ensiling reduces the pH to 3.8 to 4.2 for a good quality silage, which inhibits growth of undesirable microbes and results in an ideal preservation on the ensiled material [9]. While ensiling represent an appropriate preservation method for forages, crops and high moisture by-products, it can also result in the losses of nutrients due to undesirable fermentation process in cases where lactic acid is not adequate [10]. To overcome the nutritive losses of the ensiled material, different additives are used.

Additives are constituents that contribute to the reduction of losses, stimulate fermentation, and enrich nutritional value of silage [10]. Such additives include chemicals, enzymes, absorbents and microbial inoculants [11]. Chemical additives such as propionic acid, formic acid, sulphuric acid have been applied to high moisture (> 70% moisture) forages during ensiling for some decades. However, their use in silage is limited due to their toxic nature if not properly applied [10]. Enzymes such as xylanase, cellulase etc. are usually added to forage at ensiling to partially degrade fibre to fermentable water-soluble carbohydrates (WSC) that are consumed by lactic acid bacteria (LAB). The LAB can use fibre as source of energy to produce lactic acid [12]. The use of microbial inoculants ensures rapid and efficient fermentation of WSC to lactic acid and further predicts the adequacy of silage fermentation [13]. Lactic acid bacterial inoculants have been introduced some decades as one of microbial additives that improve forage fermentation, aerobic stability of silage and silage utilization by ruminants [14]. The most commonly LAB inoculants are obligate homofermentative, obligate heterofermentative and facultative heterofermentative LAB [15].

However, it should be noted that the addition of LAB inoculants to forage of low WSC (< 30 g/kg) content, could result to poor fermentation of the forage [16]. Haigh and Parker [17] concluded that WSC content as low as 30 g/kg may be sufficient for a stable fermentation where an effective additive is added during ensiling. In many instances, a source of readily fermentable substrate for LAB is included with commercial bacterial inoculants.

Given that LAB inoculants have been used as silage additives for a long time, their utilization is however more prominent on the ensiling of forages/crops. However, research on the use of LAB inoculants during the ensiling of high moisture by-products is limited. The present study therefore reviewed the use of microbial inoculants on high moisture by-products with special emphasis on silage fermentation and aerobic stability and livestock performance.

2. Addition of high-moisture by-products to improve the ensiling of forages

High moisture by-products such as those from the fruit juice processing contains soluble sugar that can benefit silage making from low sugar forages such as alfalfa. For example, sugar beet pulp [18] and apple pomace [19] contain WSC of 26% and 12% respectively, can be used to improve the fermentation characteristics of silage from low sugar forages. Ke et al. [20] ensiled wilted alfalfa with or without pomaces (i.e. grape and apple) and reported a reduction in silage pH, reduced proteolysis and increased lactic acid production compared to the untreated silage. In contrast, pomace addition reduced silage aerobic stability compared to the untreated silage. Fang et al. [21] added

By-products	Absorbent	Mixture (g/kg DM)		Fermentation response	Aerobic stability	Animal performance/*in vitro*	Reference
		DM	WSC				
Apple pomace	Lucerne hay (Alfalfa)	345	7.8	Improved	Reduced	ND	Ke et al. [20]
Citrus pulp	Dehydrated beet pulp	212.8	ND	Not improved	ND	ND	Megias et al. [27]
Orange pulp	Wheat straw	296.6	ND	Improved	ND	IVDMD improved	Paya et al. [28]
	Wheat straw	210.3	ND	Improved	ND	IVDMD reduced	Denek and Can [29]
Sweet potato vines	Sweet potato roots	163	ND	Not improved	ND	IVDMD reduced	Hadgu et al. [30]
Sweet potato vines	Napier grass	197	ND	Not improved	ND	ND	Kabirizi et al. [31]
Potato pulp	Dry rice	269.7	ND	Not improved	ND	ND	Zhang et al. [32]
	Dry bean straw	276.9	ND	Not improved	ND	ND	Zhang et al. [32]
	Dry maize stover	260.0	ND	Not improved	ND	ND	Zhang et al. [32]
Potato hash	Poultry litter	364.0	33.8	Not improved	Reduced	IVOMD improved	Nkosi et al. [33]
	Eragrostis curvula hay	250	22	Improved	Improved	IVOMD improved	Nkosi et al. [33]
Pineapple residue	Poultry litter	234	ND	Improved	Improved	IVOMD reduced	Nhan et al. [34]
Pineapple	Rice polishing	230	ND	Improved	Reduced	Feed intake and weight gain improved	Nhan et al. [34]
Grape pomace	Lucerne hay (alfalfa)	331	7.6	Improved			Ke et al. [20]
Wet sugar beet pulp	Dry pelleted beet pulp	907	ND	Not Improved	Reduced	IVDMD improved	Leupp et al. [35]
Tomato pomace	Ground maize grains	363	ND	Improved	ND	Feed intake improved	Galló et al. [36]
Pumpkin chopped	Dried sugar pulp	292	ND	Improved	ND	ND	Łozicki et al. [37]
	Dried sugar beet pulp	289.6	57.8	Not Improved	ND	ND	Halik et al. [38]
Banana fruit chopped	Dried sugar beet pulp	267.5	ND	Improved	ND	ND	Álvarez et al. [39]
Tomato fruit chopped	Dried sugar beet pulp	263	ND	Improved			Álvarez et al. [40]

By-products	Absorbent	Mixture (g/kg DM)		Fermentation response	Aerobic stability	Animal performance/*in vitro*	Reference
		DM	WSC				
Orange pulp	Dried citrus pulp	712	ND	Improved	Improved	IVDMD improved	Arbabi et al. [41]
	Dried sugar beet pulp	707	ND	Improved	Improved	IVDMD improved	Arbabi et al. [41]
	Wheat straw	606	ND	Improved	Improved	IVDMD improved	Arbabi et al. [41]
Apple pomace	Maize plant	213	ND	Improved	ND	IVOMD improved	Ülger et al. [42]
	Sugar beet pulp	151	ND	Improved	ND	IVOMD improved	Ülger et al. [42]
	Pumpkin pulp	115	ND	Not improved	ND	IVOMD improved	Ülger et al. [42]
Sugar beet pulp	Molassed beet pulp	186	249	Improved	Unaffected	IVDMD improved	O'Keily [43]
	Unmolassed beet pulp	188	75	Improved	ND	ND	O'Keily [43]
	Barley	189	18	Improved	ND	ND	O'Keily [43]
Citrus pulp	Wheat bran	124	ND	Improved	Reduced	OMD improved	Kordi and Naserian [44]

ND: Not detected; IVOMD, in vitro organic matter digestibility.

Table 1.
Effects of the use of absorbents on fermentation characteristics, aerobic stability and in vitro/ animal performance fed silage from high moisture plant by-products.

0, 5, 10 and 20% apple pomace in a total mixed ration that was ensiled for 90 days, and reported an increased silage ethanol production with the 20% inclusion of apple pomace. This was attributed to the increased sugar content of the silage mixture.

3. Use of absorbents to improve the ensiling of high moisture plant by-products

One of the major setbacks in ensiling agro-industrial by-products is their high moisture contents (>25%) that requires the by-products to be dehydrated or mixed with absorbents to improve the dry matter contents, compaction and ensiling process [22]. When silage DM content is less than 300 g/kg, conditions for clostridial activity are favourable, resulting in high losses and silage of low nutritional value [23]. To enhance the fermentation process and sustain nutritional quality during ensiling, various additives such as feedstuffs, nutrients and absorbents [24, 25], and non-protein nitrogen agents, chemicals and enzymes have been used [26].

High moisture by-products such as pulps and pomaces are difficult to ensile and may lead to seepages, causing nutrient losses. These by-products are usually ensiled with absorbents (i.e. dry sources) to improve both the dry matter and fermentation. The effects of adding various absorbents to high moisture by-products at ensiling are shown in **Table 1**. Adding absorbents to high moisture plant by-products at ensiling improved the fermentation (66%), silage aerobic stability (50%) and in vitro or animal performance by 74% of the responses. This variation in responses depends on the nutritive values and WSC content of the absorbents used. Nkosi et al. [45] ensiled potato hash with either *Eragrostis curvula* hay and poultry litter as absorbents. They reported higher crude protein content in the silage produced with poultry litter than that produced with the grass hay. Migwi et al. [46] ensiled citrus pulp with either straw or poultry litter and reported improved silage fermentation dynamics with these two absorbents. The addition of straw to the beet pulp improved the DM content, WSC, *in vitro* dry matter digestibility (IVDMD) and increased the fibre fraction of the silage compared to the control. Megias et al. [27] and Paya et al. [28] reported that hay and wheat straw improved silage fermentation when used as absorbent in citrus pulp silage. Islam et al. [47] reported that wheat bran and wheat straw did not improve silage fermentation when used as absorbent in apple pomace silage. Zhang et al. [32] further reported that dry rice; dry beans and dry corn stover did not improve silage fermentation when used as silage absorbent when ensiling potato pulp. Khattab et al. [48] ensiled banana wastes mixed with wheat straw and broiler litter. The silage was treated with either diluted molasses or sweet whey as nutrient (sugars) additives, which improved growth performance of buffaloes. The addition of *Eragrostis curvula* hay as an absorbent did not improve the quality of the potato hash silage [49]. Álvarez et al. [40] ensiled tomato fruit mixed with either dehydrated beet pulp or cereal straw and reported improved nutrient content in silage mixed with dehydrated beet pulp. Hadjipanayiotou [50] added either poultry litter or straw to tomato pulp silage and reported greater CP content in silage treated with poultry littler compared to the straw treated silage.

4. Use of microbial inoculants during the ensiling of high moisture by-products

4.1 Microbial inoculants

Microbial inoculants are products that are added or inoculated to forages to increase the number of microbes (e.g. LAB) in the forage at ensiling and influence the fermentation process of the forage in the silo [51]. The forage at ensiling is generally dominated by aerobic micro-organisms or facultative aerobes, with less population of LAB [52]. Forages are usually inoculated with homofermentative and facultative heterofermentative LAB to enhance LA fermentation of forages. Homofermentative LAB produces 2 moles of lactic acid from one mole of glucose, and these products contain strains species such as *Lactobacillus* (e.g. planturum, pediococcus species, and enterococcus species) [52] and the recent meta-analysis by Oliviera et al. [53] showed *Lactobacillus planturum* as the mostly used species. Heterofermenters produces one mole of lactic acid, one mole of carbon dioxide and one mole of acetic acid [52]. Homofermentative LAB are reported to yield high DM recovery and little energy loss from the silage while the heterofermentative LAB results in high DM losses, increase in silage pH and volatile fatty acids such as acetic and propionic acids [54]. According to Avila et al. [55] facultative heterofermentative LAB strains are not good for producing sugarcane silages due to increased DM losses. However, inoculation of forages with heterofermentative LAB increase the concentration of acetic acid or propionic acid, which are suitable for yeast control because of their fungicidal effect [56]. This means that heterofermentative LAB inoculants improve the aerobic stability of silage while it can be reduced with Homofermentative LAB inoculation [51, 57]. According to Muck [52] the rumen bacteria ferment lactic acid whereas acetic acid is a product of rumen fermentation. Hence there are benefits to rumen microbial growth from producing lactic acid from the silo during ensiling of forages. In a recent meta-analysis on the inoculation rates of LAB to forages, the 10^6 colony forming units (CFU)/g was common, and the 10^5 and 10^6 cfu/g inoculation rates were most effective for improving silage fermentation, reducing acetic acid production and improving DM recovery [53]. This study further reported that the recommended inoculation rate for silage inoculants varies by region, with 10^5 cfu/g being common in the United States, 10^6 cfu/g in Europe, and 10^4 cfu/g being common in some Asian and South American countries. The type of forage was the most consistent factor affecting the silage quality response to LAB inoculation [53]. With cereal grain forages such as corn, the lack of response with LAB inoculation is probably because these forages contained sufficient WSC, epiphytic bacterial population and low buffering capacity.

4.2 Silage fermentation characteristics

Bouillant and Crolbois first adopted the principle of microbial inoculation in 1909 when they applied LAB inoculants to beet pulp to improve fermentation [58]. Later in 1934, Rushmann and Meyer (1979, were cited by [59]) documented that the rate of acidification during silage fermentation is dependent on epiphytic bacteria found on forages. Currently, there are several silage inoculants available on the market with inoculation rate that ranges between 10^4 and 10^6 colony forming unit (CFU)/g [60]. Most commercially available inoculants contain homofermentative LABs, which are fast and efficient producers of lactic acid, and thus improve the silage fermentation. However, these LAB inoculants are mostly designed/produced to be used in the ensiling of forages to ensure enough LAB inoculation at ensiling. Most studies (e.g. [61, 62]) showed an increased in LAB population when LAB inoculants were applied to forages at ensiling. The response to LAB and enzyme inoculation to various high moisture by-products at ensiling are presented in **Table 2**. Literature shows that the response to LAB inoculation to forage varies a lot. Some reported positive effects in the terms of fermentation dynamics while some reported lack of response. LAB inoculation to high moisture by-products at ensiling have underwent the same pattern as with the forages. For instance, Parigi-Bini et al. [68] found that the inoculation of lactobacilli (*Lactobacillus plantarum* and

By-Product	Treatment			Fermentation	LAB type	Inoculation rate	Ensiling days	Reference
	Parameter	Control	Inoculant					
Sugar beet pulp	pH	3.91	3.95	Not improved	*L. fermentum nrrl b-4524*	-	90	Zheng et al. [63]
	LA	33	28.92	Not Improved		-		
	AA	34.69	35.07	Not Improved		-		
Tomato pomace	pH	4.97	4.57	Not Improved	Sill All	10^5 CFU g^{-1} diluted with 2L water	70	Galló et al. [36]
	LA	17.9	20.5	Not Improved				
	AA	9.16	14.2	Not Improved				
Sweet potato vines	pH	4.06	3.84	Improved	*(Lactobacillus buchneri, Lactobacillus plantarum and Entrococcus faecium)*	1.1×10^{11} CFU/g		Yacout et al. [64]
	LA	47.1	51.3	Improved				
	AA	31.7	33.2	Improved				
Orange pulp	pH	3.8	3.5	Improved	*Lactobacillus Plantarum*	1 g/kg diluted with 50 ml water (700000 U/kg)	90	Paya et al. [28]
	LA	36.4	47.2	Improved				
	AA	9.5	6.85	Not Improved				
Potato hash	pH	3.5	3.14	Improved	Viscozyme® (hemicellulose and pectinase from *Aspergillus spp*)	100 ml enzyme diluted with 1 l of water	90	Nkosi et al. [45] Mutavhatsindi et al. [65]
	LA	58.3	71.7	Improved				
	AA	6.3	3.4	Improved				
	pH	3.8	3.7	Improved	Enzymes (celluclast)	-		
	LA	36.42	41.25	Improved				
	AA	9.50	14.47	Improved				

By-Product	Treatment			Fermentation	LAB type	Inoculation rate	Ensiling days	Reference
	Parameter	Control	Inoculant					
Potato pulp	pH	3.97	3.94	Improved	Rhizopus oryzae	1×10^6 CFU g^{-1}	40	Okine et al. [66]
	LA	24.6	26.8	Improved				
	AA	10.6	12.6	Improved				
	pH	3.97	3.95	Improved	Amylomyces rouxii	1×10^6 CFU g^{-1}		
	LA	24.6	24.8	Improved				
	AA	10.6	10.0	Improved				
Peach pomace TMR	pH	4.29	4.24	Not Improved	*Pediococcus acidilactici, Lactobacillus buchneri*	- 3×10^5 CFU g^{-1}	56	Hu et al. [18]
	LA	71.1	62.1	Not Improved				
	AA	13.8	9.0	Not Improved				
Potato hash TMR	pH	4.3	4.1	Improved	Lalsil fresh	-	90	Nkosi et al. [67]
	LA	61.0	69.8	Improved		-		
	AA	31.8	36.3	Improved				
Pumpkin chopped	pH	3.96	3.78	Improved	Bacterial-enzyme- *Lactobacillus plantarum*	2×10^9 CFU g^{-1}	70	Łozicki et al. [37]
	LA	56.4	64.3	Improved				

Table 2.
Effects of LAB inoculation on fermentation of high moisture plant by-products silage.

Streptococcus) to pressed sugar beet pulp did not affect the nutritional value and fermentation of the silage. Similarly, Okine et al. [66] ensiled a daikon by-product with or without *L. plantarum* and reported no effect on fermentation characteristics of the silage. In contrast, Okine et al. [69] ensiled potato pulp with bacterial inoculants (*Lactobacillus rhamnosus*) alone, *Rhizopus oryzae* alone and their combinations, and reported reduced content of the main carbohydrates, starch and pectin in the pulp with bacterial inoculation. **Table 2** shows that 63% of the responses in this review were positive towards LAB inoculation to high moisture by-products at ensiling.

4.3 Aerobic stability of silage

The aerobic stability is a term that nutritionists have used to define the length of time that silage remains cool and does not spoil after it is exposed to air [70]. The aerobic deterioration of silage may increase the risk of proliferation of potential pathogenic or undesirable microorganisms thus affecting the performance of animals fed the silage. In most cases, aerobic deterioration of silage happens with silages that contain high residual sugars [14]. It is noteworthy that *Lactobacillus buchneri* (LB), a heterofermentative LAB inoculant [51, 57] have been reported to improve the aerobic stability of silages due to increased acetic acid production. Previous research with potato hash silage [49, 71] showed improved aerobic stability of silage with LB inoculation. Li et al. [72] ensiled a mixture of corn steep liquor with wheat straw and treated with either heterofermentative or homofermentative LAB. They reported an increase in acetic acid content and improved aerobic stability of silage with heterofermentative LAB compared to untreated silage. The inoculation of LB during the ensiling of forages is often criticised due to increase in silage pH, acetic acid and losses in DM and energy [12, 15, 56, 73–80]. However, if aerobic stability is improved, the loss of nutrients incurred by the addition of LB may be moderate in comparison with what might have been lost at feed out through aerobic deterioration [71].

5. Effects of microbial inoculation to ensiled totally mixed rations (TMRs) on fermentation and aerobic stability

Due to the high moisture content in fresh high moisture by-products, it is more advantageous to mix them with other dry feed materials before ensiling. This technique helps to omit the time of mixing before feeding, minimize the risk of effluent production and avoids self-selection of feeds by animals [81, 82]. In some studies, TMRs that contained high moisture by-products (e.g. [83]) [49] were formulated and ensiled. Nkosi and Meeske [71] reported an improved silage fermentation, aerobic stability and animal growth performance when TMR that contained potato hash was treated with LAB inoculant. However, Nishino and Hattori [83] reported improved silage fermentation but LAB inoculation was not worth in the aerobic stability of TMR silage. This might be attributed to the addition of various feed ingredients that might have helped to stabilize the TMR silage.

6. Animal performance

The production of silage will not be worth if it is rejected by animals during the feeding out phase. Animal performance includes feed intake, feed palatability, nutrient digestion, daily gains, milk and meat production. The results on the performance of animals fed plant by-product silage treated with LAB varies like when animals are fed LAB treated silages from plants/forages. According to **Table 3**,

By-products	LAB type	Inoculation rate	Animal species/*in vitro*	Response	Reference
Potato hash	Bonsilage forte (*Lactobacillus paracasei*, *Lactobacillus lactis*, *Pediococcus acidilactici* and Lalsil Fresh LB (*Lactobacillus buchneri*)	2.5×10^5 CFU g^{-1}	Mutton Merino rams	Improved gross energy, crude protein and fibre digestibility. Improved nitrogen intake and retention.	Nkosi et al. [49]
Spent mushroom substrate	Mixture of *Enterobacter ludwigii* KU201-3, *Bacillus cereus* KU206-3, *Bacillus subtilis* KU3, *Bacillus subtilis* KU201-7, *Saccharomyces cerevisiae*, and *Lactobacillus plantarum*	1×10^9 CFU g^{-1}	Cross bred rams	Improved EE digestibility and nitrogen retention.	Seok et al. [84]
Spent mushroom substrate	*Enterobacter ludwigii* KU201-3, *Bacillus cereus* KU206-3, *Bacillus subtilis* KU3, *Saccharomyces cerevisiae, and Lactobacillus plantarum*	Each strain at 0.12% v/w	Hanwoo steers	Improved ADG, FCR and FI	Kim et al. [85]
Tomato pomace	Sil All 4x4 (*Enterococcus faecium, Pediococcus acidilactici, Lactobacillus plantarum, Lactobacillus salivarius)*	1×10^5 CFU g^{-1}	Game	Improved	Galló et al. [36]
Sugar beet pulp	Sil add *(Lactobacillus plantarum, Pediococcus acidilactici, Streptococcus bovis and Selenomonas ruminantium)*	0.5 g/kg FM basis	Hereford and Friesian steers	Unaffected	O'Keily [43]
Chinese cabbage	*Lactobacillus plantarum*	5 mg/kg FM basis	*In vitro*	Increased DM digestibility.	Cao et al. [7]
Cabbage waste	Silobac® (*lactobacillus plantarum* and *Pediococcus pentosaceus*)	5×10^5 CFU g^{-1}	*In vitro*	Increased DM digestibility.	De Rezende et al. [86]
Yacon (*Smallanthus sonchifolius*)	Chikuso-1 (*lactobacillus plantarum*)	5 mg/kg FM basis	*In vitro*	Increased DM digestibility.	Wang et al. [82]
Avocado pulp	Emsilage® and Sil-All®	3.5×10^5 CFU g^{-1}	*In Vitro*	Improved silage degradation	Nkosi et al. [87]

Table 3.
Effects of microbial inoculation to high moisture plant by-product silage on animal growth performance.

LAB inoculation to high moisture plant by-products improved animal performance in almost all the literature consulted, except for the sugar beet pulp silage reported by O'Keily [43]. It is well known that improved performance by animals fed LAB treated silages are difficult to explain [26]. However, Weinberg et al. [88] suggested that the interaction of LAB and rumen microbes and the alteration of LAB and rumen fermentation might be attributed to the improvement of animal performance with LAB treated silages.

Inoculation of potato hash silage with *L. buchneri* did not change the DM or organic matter (OM), but bonsilage forte inoculation improved digestibility of ether extract and increased nitrogen (N) intake and retention in sheep fed the silage [49]. Further, Thomas et al. [89] compared the effects of two bacterial inoculants on digestibility, growth performance and carcass characteristics of growing pigs fed the ensiled potato hash, and reported no improvement with LAB inoculation on the growth performance and meat characteristics of growing pigs. Okine et al. [69] ensiled potato pulp with *L. rhamnosus* and *Rhizopus oryzae,* and reported lack of influence from LAB inoculation on the digestibility of the silage by ruminants. In contrast, Li et al. [72] treated corn steep liquor silage with LAB and reported improved DM digestibility, which resulted in less methane production compared to untreated silage. Further, a study by Pulido et al. [90] showed an improvement in the nutritive value of sugar beef pulp silage with LAB inoculation, which increased milk production from dairy cows by 2%, though milk composition was not affected by the inoculation.

Methane, a greenhouse gas produced from enteric fermentation in the rumen, is a major concern in ruminant production globally. It is well indicated that by improving forage quality and digestibility, this gas production can be reduced. In terms of reduction gas production with LAB inoculation, very few studies have tested this effect in silages from high moisture by-products. Cao et al. [7] reported a reduced gas production with *L. plantarum* inoculated to vegetable residue silage, which suggest that LAB inoculation can be effective in reducing gas emission in silages. However, Ellis et al. [91] have cautioned that LAB inoculation to forage will not always give positive response. They mentioned that the strain and dose differences, different basal silages and ensiling conditions might be responsible for the variability in responses from LAB inoculation.

7. Properties required in high moisture plant by-products for efficient silage fermentation

As indicated earlier, the low DM content in high moisture plant by-products is a concern since it can promote a clostridial type of fermentation if not improved prior to ensiling. According to Muck [52], most silages are produced at DM content that ranges from 300 to 500 g/kg, hence the DM of these by-products should be increased. This can be achieved by mixing with absorbents/dry forages. Also, the success of ensiling is determined by various factors that include the anaerobic conditions in the silo, WSC content, the buffering capacity of the pre-ensiled forage, and the epiphytic bacteria. Bacterial inoculation will be worthless if the by-products contain insufficient sugars, which should be consumed by LAB to produce lactic acid, which will reduce silage pH and preserve the crop [23].

8. Conclusion

Good quality silage can be produced from high moisture plant by-products with or without LAB inoculation. Increasing the DM content of high moisture plant by-products to >30% is required for efficient fermentation. It should be noted that there are no specific LAB inoculants designed for inoculation to high moisture plant by-products. The efficacy of LAB inoculation to forages depends highly on the type of crop/by-product, the strain and different doses and the ensiling management.

Author details

Bhutikini D. Nkosi[1,2*], Cyprial N. Ncobela[1], Ronald S. Thomas[1], Ingrid M.M. Malebana[1], Francuois Muller[1], Sergio Álvarez[3] and Robin Meeske[4]

1 Agricultural Research Council: Animal Production Institute, Irene, South Africa

2 Centre for Sustainable Agriculture and Rural Development, University of the Free State, Bloemfontein, South Africa

3 Animal Production and Forage Research Unit, Canary Agronomic Research Institute (ICIA), La Laguna, Tenerife, Spain

4 Directorate: Animal Sciences, Department of Agriculture Western Cape, Outeniqua Research Farm, George, South Africa

*Address all correspondence to: dnkosi@arc.agric.za

References

[1] Mirzaei-Aghsaghali, A., Maheri-Sis, N., 2008. Nutritive value of some agro-industrial by-products for ruminants – a review. World J. Zool. 3, 40-46.

[2] Sindhu, A. A., Khan, M. A., Nisa, M. U., Sarwar, M., 2002. Agro-industrial by-products as a potential source of livestock feed. Int. J. Agric. Biol. 4, 307-310.

[3] Arowolo, M.A., He, J., 2018. Use of probiotics and botanical extracts to improve ruminant production in the tropics. Anim. Nutr. 4, 241-249.

[4] Jideani, A. I., Anyasi, T. A., Mchau, G. R., Udoro, E. O., Onipe, O. O., 2017. Processing and preservation of fresh-cut fruit and vegetable products. Postharvest Handling, Intech Open: London, UK, 47-73.

[5] Tufarelli, V., Laudadio, V., 2011. Effect of wheat middlings-based total mixed ration on milk production and composition responses of lactating dairy ewes. J. Dairy Sci. 94, 376-381.

[6] Charmley, E., Nelson, D., Zvomuya, F., 2006. Nutrient cycling in the vegetable processing industry: Utilization of potato by-products. Can. J. Soil. Sci. 86, 621-629.

[7] Cao, Y., Cai, Y., Takahashi, T., Yoshida, N., Tohno, M., Uegaki, R., Nonaka, K., Terada, F., 2011. Effect of lactic acid bacteria inoculant and beet pulp addition on the fermentation characteristics and in vitro ruminal digestion of vegetable residue silage. J. Dairy Sci. 94, 3902-3912.

[8] Ferreira, A. C. H., Rodriguez, N. M., Neiva, J. N. M., Pimentel, P. G., Gomes, S. P., Campos, W. E., Lopes, F. C. F., 2015. Nutritional evaluation of elephant-grass silages with different levels of by-products from the cashew juice industry. R. Bras. Zootec. 44, 434-442.

[9] Chavira, J.S., 2016. Advances in silage production in utilization. Chapter 5: Potential use of nonconventional silages in ruminant feeding for the Tropical and Subtropical areas. Pp. 85-98.

[10] Vieira, D. A., Cezário, A. S., Valente, T. N. P., Ribeiro, J. C., Santos, W. B. R., Ferreira, P. R. N., 2017. Evaluation of the addition of urea or calcium oxide (CaO) on the recovery of dry matter of the by-product of sweet corn silage. J. Agric. Sci. 9. 141-148.

[11] Yunus, M., Ohba, N., Shimojo, M., Furuse, M., Masuda, Y., 2000. Effects of adding urea and molasses on Napier grass silage quality. Asian-Australas. J. Anim. Sci. 13, 1542-1547.

[12] Xing, L., Chen, L.J., Han, L.J., 2009. The effect of an inoculant and enzymes on fermentation and nutritive value of sorghum straw silages. Bioresour. Technol. 100, 488-491.

[13] Wang, L., Guan, L., Fang, J., Cai, Y., Cao, Y., 2019. Fermentation characteristics and in vitro ruminal digestion of yacon residue silage with lactic acid bacteria inoculant or beet pulp. Rev. Bras. de Zootec. 42, 48:e20180152.

[14] Weinberg, Z.G., Ashbell, G, Hen, Y., Azriel, A., 1993. The effect of applying lactic acid bacteria on the aerobic stability of silages. J. Appl. Bacteriol. 75, 512 – 518.

[15] Bernardi, A., Härter, C.J., Silva, A.W.L., , Reis, R.A., Rabelo, C.H.S., 2019. A meta-analysis examining lactic acid bacteria inoculants for maize silage: Effects on fermentation, aerobic stability, nutritive value and livestock production. Grass Forage Sci. 74, 596-612.

[16] Seale, D. R., Henderson, A. R., Pettersson, K. O., Lowe, J. F., 1986. The effect of addition of sugar and inoculation with two commercial inoculants on the fermentation of lucerne silage in laboratory silos. Grass Forage Sci. 41, 61-70.

[17] Haigh, P. M., Parker, J. W. G., 1985. Effect of silage additives and wilting on silage fermentation, digestibility and intake, and on live weight change of young cattle. Grass Forage Sci. 40, 429-436.

[18] Hu, X., Hao, W., Wang, H., Ning, T., Zheng, M., Xu, C., 2015. Fermentation characteristics and lactic acid bacteria succession of total mixed ration silages formulated with peach pomace. Asian-Aust. J. Anim. Sci. 28, 502-510.

[19] Guler, T., Cerci, I.H., Ciftci, M., Ertas, O.N., 2006. Can apples be used as a source of fermentable carbohydrate when making alfalfa silage? Revue Med. Vet. 157, 163-167.

[20] Ke, W.C., Yang, F.Y., Undersander, D.J., Guo, X.S., 2015, Fermentation characteristics, aerobic stability, proteolysis and lipid composition of alfalfa silage ensiled with apple or grape pomace. Anim. Feed Sci. Technol. 202, 12-19.

[21] Fang, J., Cao, Y., Matsuzaki, M., Suzuki, H., 2016. Effects of apple pomace proportion levels on the fermentation quality of total mixed ration silage and its digestibility, preference and ruminal fermentation in beef cows. Anim. Sci. J. 87, 217-223.

[22] Khorvash, M., Colombatto, D., Beauchemin, K.A., Ghorbani, G.R., Samei, A., 2006. Use of absorbents and inoculants to enhance the quality of corn silage. Can. J. Anim. Sci. 86, 97 – 107.

[23] McDonald, P., Edwards, R.A., Greenhalgh, J.F.D., Morgan, C.A., Sinclair, L.A. & Wilkinson, R.G., 2010. Animal Nutrition. 7th Edition. Pearson, Prentice Hall.

[24] Charmley, E., 2001. Towards improved silage quality – a review. Can. J. Anim. Sci. 81, 157 – 168.

[25] Elferink, S. J. W. H. O., Driehuis, F., Gottschal, J. C., Spoelstra, S. F., 1999. Silage fermentation processes and their manipulation. FAO Plant Production and Protection Papers, 17-30.

[26] Muck, R.E., Nadeau, E.M.G., McAllister, T.A., Contreras-Govea, F.E., Santos, M.C., Kung Jr., L., 2018. Silage review: Recent advances and future uses of silage additives. J. Dairy Sci. 101, 3980-4000.

[27] Megias, M.D., Hernandez, F., Cano, J-A., Martinez-Teruel, J.A., 1998. Effects of different additives on the cell wall and mineral fractions of artichoke (*Cynara scolymus*) and orange (*Citrus aurantium L.*) by product silage. J. Sci. Food Agric. 76, 173-178.

[28] Paya, H., Taghizadeh, A., Lashkari, S., 2015. Effects of Lactobacillus plantarum and hydrolytic enzymes on fermentation and ruminal degradability of orange pulp silage. J. Biosci. Biotechnol. 4, 349-357.

[29] Denek, N., Can, A., 2007. Effect of wheat straw and different additives on silage quality and In vitro dry matter digestibility of wet orange pulp. J. Anim. Vet. Adv. 6, 217-219.

[30] Hadgu, G. Z., Negesse, T., Nurfeta, A., 2015. Nutritive value of fresh dried (hay) and ensiled vines of four sweet potato (*Ipomoea batatas*) varieties grown in southern Ethiopia. Trop. Subtrop. Agroecosystems. 18, 195-205.

[31] Kabirizi, J. M., Lule, P. M., Lutwama, V., Kigongo, J., Isabirye, D., 2016. Training Report: Training of trainers and farmers' training on validated sweet potato silage making

and use in Masaka and Kamuli districts. Pp 1-40.

[32] Zhang, W. W., Zhang, Y. G., Liu, Z., 2012. Effect of different absorbents on fermentation quality of wet potato pulp. Anim Vet Adv. 11, 4230-4235.

[33] Nkosi, B. D., Vadlani, P. V., Brijwani, K., Nanjunda, A., Meeske, R., 2012. Effects of bacterial inoculants and an enzyme on the fermentation quality and aerobic stability of ensiled whole-crop sweet sorghum. S. Afr. J. Anim. Sci. 42, 232-240.

[34] Nhan, N.T.H., van Hon, N., Preston, T.R., 2009. Ensiling with or without additives to preserve pineapple residue and reduce pollution of the environment. Livest. Res. Rural Developm. 21:7.

[35] Leupp, J.L., Encinias, A.M., Bauer, M.L., Caton, J.S., Gilbery, T.C., Carlson, J., Lardy, G.P., 2006. Ensiling properties of wet sugar beet pulp and the addition of liquid feedstuffs or urea. J. Sugar Beet Res. 43, 85-97.

[36] Galló, J., Fernye, C., Orosz, S., Katona, K., Szemethy, L., 2017. Tomato pomace silage as a potential new supplementary food for game species. Agric. Food Sci. 26, 79-89.

[37] Łozicki, A., Koziorzębska, A., Halik, G., Dymnicka, M., Arkuszewska, E., Niemiec, T., Bogdan, J., 2015. Effect of ensiling pumpkin (*Cucurbita maxima D.*) with dried sugar beet pulp on the content of bioactive compounds in silage and its antioxidant potential. Anim. Feed Sci. Technol. 206, 108-113.

[38] Halik, G. D., Lozicki, A., Koziorzebska, A., Dymnicka, M. A. R. I. A., Arkuszewska, E., 2014. Effect of ensiling pumpkin Cucurbita maxima with the addition of inoculant or without it on chemical composition and quality of silages. Annals of Warsaw University of Life Sciences-SGGW. Anim. Sci. 53. 103-110.

[39] Álvarez, S., Mendez, P., Martinez-Fernandez, A., 2015. Fermentative and nutritive quality of banana by-product silage for goats. J. Appl. Anim. Res. 43, 396-401.

[40] Álvarez, S., Martínez-Fernández, A., Méndez P., 2020. Ensiling potential of fresh tomato waste with dehydrated beet pulp and cereal straw as additives. Anim. Nutr. Feed Technol. 20, 381-392.

[41] Arbabi, S., Ghoorchi, T., Naserian, A.A., 2008. The effect of dried citrus pulp, dried beet sugar pulp and wheat Straw as silage additives on by-products of orange silage. Asian J. Anim. Sci. 2, 35-42.

[42] Ülger, I., Kaliber, M., Ayaşan, T., Küçük, O., 2018. Chemical composition, organic matter digestibility and energy content of apple pomace silage and its combination with corn plant, sugar beet pulp and pumpkin pulp. S. Afr. J. Anim. Sci. 48, 497 – 503.

[43] O'Keily, P. 1992. The effects of ensiling sugarbeet pulp with grass on silage composition, effluent production and animal performance. Irish J. Agric. Food Rese. 31, 115-128.

[44] Kordi, M., Naserian, A.A., 2012. Influence of wheat bran as a silage additive on chemical composition, in situ degradability and in vitro gas production of citrus pulp silage. Afr. J. Biotechnol. 11, 12669-12674.

[45] Nkosi, B.D., Meeske, R., Langa, T., Motiang, M.D., Mutavhatsindi, T.F., Thomas, R.S., Groenewald, I.B., Baloyi, J.J., 2015. The influence of ensiling potato hash waste with enzyme/bacterial inoculant mixtures on the fermentation characteristics, aerobic stability and nutrient digestion of the resultant silage by rams. Small Rumin. Res. 127, 28-35.

[46] Migwi, P.K., Gallagher, J.R., van Barneveld, R.J., 2001. The nutritive

value of citrus pulp ensiled with wheat straw and poultry litter for sheep. Austr. J. Experim. Agric. 41, 1143-1148.

[47] Islam, S., Islam, M. N., Matsuzaki, M., 2014. Apple pomace silage ethanol intake and its effect on sheep. Bangladesh J. Anim. Sci. 43, 224-231.

[48] Khattab, H.M., Kholif, A.M., El-Alamy, H.A., Salem, F.A., El-Shewy, A.A., 2000. Ensiled banana wastes with molasses or whey for lactating buffaloes during early lactation. Asian-Aus. J. Anim. Sci. 13, 619-624.

[49] Nkosi, B. D., Meeske, R., Van Der Merwe, H. J., Groenewald, I. B., 2010. Effects of homofermentative and heterofermentative bacterial silage inoculants on potato hash silage fermentation and digestibility in rams. Anim. Feed Sci. Technol. 157, 195-200.

[50] Hadjipanayiotou, M., 1994. Laboratory evaluation of ensiled olive cake, tomato pulp and poultry litter. Livestock Res. Rural Dev. 6, 1-5

[51] Weinberg, Z.G., Muck, R.E., 1996. New trends in development and use of inoculants for silage. FEMS Microbiol. Reviews 19, 53-68.

[52] Muck, R.E, 2010a. Silage microbiology and its control through silage additives. R. Bras. Zootec. 39, 183-191.

[53] Oliveira, A.S., Weinberg, Z.G., Ogunade, I.M., Cervantes, A.A.P., Arriola, K.G., Jiang, Y., Kim, D., Li, X., Goncalves, M.C.M., Vyas, D., Adesogan, A.T., 2016. Meta-analysis of effects of inoculation with homofermentative and facultative heterofermentative lactic acid bacteria on silage fermentation, aerobic stability and performance of dairy cows. J. Dairy Sci. 100, 4587-4603.

[54] Contreras-Govea, F., Muck, R.E., 2006. Microbial inoculants for silage. Focus on Forage 8(4), 1-4.

[55] Avila, C.L.S, Carvalho, B.F., Pinto, J.C., Duarte, W.F., Schwan, R.F., 2014. The use of Lactobacillus species as cultures for enhancing the quality of sugar cane silage. J. Dairy Sci. 97, 940-951.

[56] Moon, N.J., 1983. Inhibition of the growth of acid tolerant yeasts by acetic acid, lactic acid and propionate, and their synergistic mixture. J. Appl. Bacteriol. 55, 453-460.

[57] Holzer, M.E., Mayrhuber, E., Danner, H., Braun, R., 2003. The role of Lactobacillus buchneri in forage preservation. Trends Biotechnol. 21, 282 – 287.

[58] Watson, S.T., Nash, J.M., 1960. The conservation of grass and forage crops. Oliver and Boyd, LTD, Edinburg, UK.

[59] Fish, S.L., 1991. Effect of a silage microbial inoculant on animal performance and silage digestibility. MSc thesis, Michigan State University, USA.

[60] Muck, R.E., 2010b. Silage additives and management issues. Proceedings of Idaho Alfalfa Forage Conference, Best Western Burley Inn, Burley, Idaho, USA. 16 – 17 February, pp. 49-55.

[61] Chen, J., Stokes, R.M., Wallace, C.R., 1994. Effects of enzyme-inoculant systems on preservation and nutritive value of hay crop and corn silages. J. Dairy Sci. 77, 501-512.

[62] Kung, L., Tung, R.S., Maciorowski, K., 1991. Effect of a microbial inoculant (Ecosyl™) and/or a glycopeptide antibiotic (*vancomycin*) on fermentation and aerobic stability of wilted alfalfa silage. Anim. Feed Sci. Technol. 35, 37 48.

[63] Zheng, Y., Yu, C., Cheng, Y. S., Lee, C., Simmons, C. W., Dooley, T. M., Zhang, R., Jenkins, B.M., Van der Gheynst, J. S., 2012. Integrating sugar

beet pulp storage, hydrolysis and fermentation for fuel ethanol production. Appl. Energy. 93, 168-175.

[64] Yacout, M. H., Amany, A., Khayyal, A., Shwerab, A. M., Khalel, M. S., 2016. Introduce sweet potato vines as good roughage for small ruminants. EC Vet. Sci. 2, 184-204.

[65] Mutavhatsindi, T. F., Nkosi, B. D., Baloyi, J. J., Langa, T., 2018. Effects of a fibrolytic enzyme and bacterial inoculants on the fermentation, chemical composition and aerobic stability of ensiled potato hash. S. Afr. J. Anim. Sci. 48, 244-252.

[66] Okine, A., Yimamu, A., Hanada, M., Izumita, M., Zunong, M., Okamoto, M., 2007. Ensiling characteristics of daikon (*Raphanus sativus*) by-product and its potential as an animal feed resource. Anim. Feed Sci. Technol. 136, 248-264.

[67] Nkosi, B.D., Kanengoni, A.T., Thomas, R.S., 2011. Effects of ensiling total mixed potato hash ration with or without bacterial inoculation on silage fermentation and nutritive value for growing pigs. J. Anim. Vet. Adv. 10, 1667-1672.

[68] Parigi-Bini, R., Albuzio, A., Cinetto, M., Nicaarto, G., 1991. D (−) and L (+) lactic acid in maize and pressed beet pulp silages treated with lactobacilli. Zootec. Nutr. Anim. 17, 321-326.

[69] Okine, A., Hanada, M., Aibibula, Y., Okamoto, M., 2005. Ensiling of potato pulp with or without bacterial inoculants and its effects on fermentation quality, nutrient composition and nutritive value. Anim. Feed Sci. Technol. 121, 329-343.

[70] McDonald, P. 1981. The biochemistry of silage. John Wiley and Sons, Ltd., Chichester, UK.

[71] Nkosi, B.D., Meeske, R., 2010. Effects of ensiling totally mixed potato hash ration with or without a heterofermentative bacterial inoculant on silage fermentation, aerobic stability, growth performance and digestibility in lambs. Anim. Feed Sci. Technol. 161, 38-48.

[72] Li, H., Zhang, L., Chen, L., Zhu, Q., Wang, W., Qiao, J., 2016. *Lactobacillus acidophilus* alleviates the inflammatory response to *enterotoxigenic Escherichia coli K88* via inhibition of the NF- κ B and p38 mitogen-activated protein kinase signaling pathways in piglets. BMC Microbiol. 16, 1-8.

[73] Reich, L.J. and Kung, L. Jr., 2010. Effects of combining Lactobacillus buchneri 40788 with various lactic acid bacteria on the fermentation and aerobic stability of corn silage. Anim. Feed Sci. Technol. 159, 105-109.

[74] Wilkinson, J. M., Davies, D. R., 2013. The aerobic stability of silage: key findings and recent developments. Grass Forage Sci. 68, 1-19.

[75] Álvarez, S., Méndez, P., Fresno, M., 2016. Ensilado de suero de quesería para alimentación animal (*Ensilage of cheese whey for animal feed*). Instituto Canario de Investigaciones Agrarias. Tenerife, Spain. Pp. 8.

[76] Muck, R.E., Kung Jr., L., 1997. Effects of silage additives on ensiling. Proc. Silage: Field to Feedbunk. North America Conference. NRAES-99. Northeast Regional Agricultural Engineering Service, Ithaca, NY. Page 187-199.

[77] Nguyen, T. A. H., Ngo, H. H., Guo, W. S., Zhang, J., Liang, S., Yue, Q. Y., Li, Q., Nguyen, T. V., 2013. Applicability of agricultural waste and by-products for adsorptive removal of heavy metals from wastewater. Bioresour. Technol. 148, 574-585.

[78] Nkosi, B. D., Groenewald, I. B., Meeske, R., Motiang, M. D., Langa, T.,

2013. Effects of inoculating citrus (*Citrus sinensis*) tree leaves with either bacterial or whey on the fermentation and aerobic stability of silage. Afr. J. Agric. Res. 8, 792-796.

[79] O'Keily, P. 1991. A note on the influence of five absorbents on silage composition and effluent retention in small-scale silos. Irish J. Agric. Res. 30, 153-158.

[80] Živkov-Baloš M., Jakšić S., Mihaljev Ž., Obradović S., Ljubojević D., Stojanov I., Jovičin M., 2014. Nutritive value of vitaminized silages. XVI International Symposium, Feed Technology held in the Institute of Food Technology, University of Novi Sad, Serbia, 30 October, pp. 28.

[81] Nishino, N., Hirada, H., Sakaguchi, Ei., 2003. Evaluation of fermentation and aerobic stability of wet brewers grains ensiled alone or in combination with various feeds as a total mixed ration. J. Sci. Food Agric. 83, 557-563.

[82] Wang, F., Nishino, N., 2008. Effect of aerobic exposure after silo opening on feed intake and digestibility of total mixed ration silage containing wet brewers grains or soybean curd residue. Grassl. Sci. 54, 164-166.

[83] Nishino, N, Hattori, H., 2007. Resistance to aerobic deterioration of total mixed ration silage inoculated with and without homofermentative or heterofermentative lactic acid bacteria. J. Sci. Food Agric. 87, 2420 – 2426.

[84] Seok, J.S., Kim, Y.I., Lee, Y.H, Choi, D. Y., Kwak, W.S., 2016. Effect of feeding a by-product feed-based silage on nutrients intake, apparent digestibility, and nitrogen balance in sheep. J. Anim. Sci. Technol. 58, 9. https://doi.org/10.1186/s40781-016-0091-7.

[85] Kim, Y., Seok, J-S., Kwak, W.S., 2015. Evaluation of microbially ensiled spent mushroom (*Pleurotus osteratus*) substrates (bed-type cultivation) as a roughage for ruminants. J. Anim. Sci. Technol. 52, 117-124.

[86] De Rezende, A.V., Rabelo, C.H.S., da Silva, M.R.M., Harter, C.J., Veiga, R.M., 2015. Wasted cabbage (Brassica oleracea) silages treated with different levels of ground corn and silage inoculant. Rev. Bras. Zootec. 44, 296-302.

[87] Nkosi, B.D., Meeske, R., Muya, M.C., Langa, T., Thomas, R.S., Malebana, I.M.M., Motiang, M.D., van Niekerk, J.A., 2020. Microbial additives affect silage quality and ruminal dry matter degradability of avocado (*Persia Americana*) pulp silage. S. Afr. J. Anim. Sci. 49, 997-1007.

[88] Weinberg, Z.G., Muck, R.E., Weimer, P.J., 2003. The survival of silage inoculant lactic acid bacteria in rumen fluid. J. Appl. Microbiol. 94, 1066-1071.

[89] Thomas, R., Nkosi, B.D., Umesiobi, D., Meeske, R., Kanengoni, A.T., Langa, T., 2010. Evaluation of potato hash silage from two bacterial inoculants and their effects on the growth performance of grower pigs. S. Afr. J. Anim. Sci. 40, 488 - 490.

[90] Pulido, R., Garcia, E., Beltrain, I., Daza, J., Keim, J., Castillo, I., 2020. Effect of a homofermentative lactic acid bacteria additive on the quality of sugar-beet pulp silage and animal response of dairy cows with restricted access to pasture. Chilean J. Agric. Res. 80, 234-240.

[91] Ellis, J.L., Hindrichsen, I.K., Klop, G., Kinley, R.D., Milora, N., Bannink, A., Dijkstra, J., 2016. Effects of lactic acid bacteria silage inoculation on methane emission and productivity of Holstein Friesian dairy cattle. J. Dairy Sci. 99, 7159-7174.

Chapter 8

Incorporating Silages into Preweaned Dairy Calf Diets

Sylvia I. Kehoe, Paweł Górka and Zhijun J. Cao

Abstract

Supplementing forage to preweaned calves has shown some positive effects, such as stabilization of the rumen environment, limiting abnormal behaviors, and increasing starter intake. However, dry forages can be limited and cost prohibitive in some areas of the world. Contrastingly, ensiled forages are commonly found on most dairy farms and are low cost. Therefore, the objective of this review was to focus specifically on ensiled forages and how they affect preweaned calves. There are few studies that have focused on providing ensiled forages and most of them have used corn silage. Although impacts on rumen development and nutrient digestibility have been variable, feed intake and efficiency were not affected in most reviewed studies. Growth and health parameters were also either not affected or improved. Therefore, with careful silage feeding management, the supplementation of ensiled feeds may be used to provide similar benefits of dry forages to preweaned dairy calves.

Keywords: rumen development, forage, digestibility, feed intake, performance

1. Introduction

Ensiled feeding has become more common around the world and is becoming an active area of calf nutrition research. So far, thorough reviews have been published on the effects of different feed type exposure to dairy calves, including the influence of forage feeding on rumen development, growth rate, feeding behavior, and many other factors in young calves [1, 2]. Also, an excellent meta-analysis on the effects of forage provision to dairy calves is available in the literature [3]. In this meta-analysis, 27 studies were evaluated and the authors found an increase in starter feed intake, average daily gain (ADG), body weight (BW) and modulation of ruminal fermentation when forage sources were offered to preweaned calves. But they also found a decrease in feed efficiency (FE) when calves were offered alfalfa hay (AH) in addition to grain based starter feed. An important conclusion from those reviews is that there are multiple interactions between the type of starter, the forage source, and the amount of forage offered, thereby, not allowing any simple guidelines to be offered to dairy farmers. Although those reviews provide excellent information on forage feeding to preweaned calves, this chapter is designed to focus specifically on ensiled forages in preweaned calf diets.

Feedstuffs for calves are separated into two categories: liquid and solid feeds. Liquid feed is either milk or milk replacer and provides the main source of nutrients for the growing calf until its gastrointestinal tract and rumen become developed enough to transition to solid feed. The solid feed is usually a grain of some kind, either whole, processed, or pelleted, with or without a forage source. The addition of solid feed to the calf's diet should be done early in life to promote the development of the calf's rumen [1, 4]. However, the individual ingredients in solid feed for calf diets have been a hot research topic since the 1950s and earlier. As dairy production has progressed scientifically with more data and research available, farmers have struggled to keep up with current recommendations, including feeding forage sources. Therefore, calf feeding recommendations, in terms of forage supplementation, differ depending on the geographical region. Some countries, such as the United States (US), generally recommend that dairy calves are not fed forage before weaning [5]. Other countries, such as those located within the European Union (EU), recommend that these pre-ruminants are provided with a forage source, as also indicated by numerous studies on feeding forage to calves conducted in EU and their results being widely propagated in EU [6, 7], but that feeding forage can be also avoided e.g. by including whole grain in starter feed [8–10].

In a survey of eleven dairy farms in South East England, two farms supplemented hay, two supplemented silage, four supplemented straw, and three supplemented with no forage to calves [11]. The age of calves or method of forage supplementation was not described but it is concluded to be more common to provide than not to provide forage to calves in South East England. In the US, a nationwide survey indicated small farms (30–99 lactating cows) begin providing calves with forage at 31.5 days of age, medium farms (100–999 lactating cows) at 43.1 days of age, and large farms (1,000 or more) at 58.1 days of age. The forage type was not described. However, it is evident that in the US, smaller farms provide forage earlier than larger farms. In Canada, farms possessing automatic calf feeders offered hay more commonly (93% of farms) than farms using manual calf feeding (66% of farms). Age for access to hay was as early as 5–7 days and access to a total mixed ration (TMR), usually a silage based feed mix, as early as 15–30 days of age for both types of calf feeding systems [12]. An Australian farm survey reported 64% of farms allowed calves access to roughage at less than 1 week of age, 23% at 2 weeks of age, and 13% at 3 or more weeks of age. Of those farms, 62% offered hay, 23% offered straw, 13% offered hay and straw, and 2% offered grass only [13]. All of these studies support substantial differences between geographical regions in terms of feeding forages to preweaned dairy calves.

The evaluation of using ensiled feeds to enhance calf gain and health needs to be reviewed purposefully, as a separate component from dry forages. Feeding dry forages, such as hay or straw, has been reported to improve calf performance in numerous studies (as summarized, for example, by [1] or [3]); however, these dried forages, especially AH, may be difficult and expensive to obtain in certain parts of the world. Contrastingly, most farms throughout the world have some ensiled feed present on the farm that could be an easy potential feedstuff to supplement calf diets. Silages are usually staple ingredients in a lactating cow ration and, therefore, accessible and less costly than dried forages. However, based on aforementioned reports of forage feeding to calves in commercial settings [11–13] and available literature reviews [1–3], a usage of silages in diets for preweaned calves is not very common. The objective of this review is to summarize available research to determine whether ensiled forages can be considered as a valuable forage source in calf diets.

2. Why is forage important for young calves?

Although dairy calves grow and mature into functional ruminants, they are born with an underdeveloped rumen [4, 14]. These pre-ruminants need to be cared for in a way that will help develop their rumen function as well as provide them nutrients for growth and development. A smooth transition from liquid to solid feed can be accomplished by providing a good quality solid feed alongside adequate levels of milk [1, 4]. However, the parameters for what constitutes good quality solid feed are variable, depending on the research study and the nutritionist.

Despite aforementioned discrepancies on specific recommendations for solid feed composition, it is widely accepted that concentrates, and particularly cereal grains, should be the most important ingredient of solid feed offered to dairy calves [1, 4]. This is due to the stimulatory impact of early intake of cereal grains on rumen epithelium development in calves. Compared to consumption of forages which mainly provide cellulose and hemicellulose, consumption of cereal grains which are abundant in starch, results in greater concentrations of propionate and butyrate in the rumen, in expense of acetate [15, 16]. Both propionate, and especially butyrate, are the most potent stimulators of ruminal epithelial cell proliferation [17, 18]. Thus, early intake of cereal grains by calves translates into faster ruminal papillae growth and greater surface area for nutrient absorption early in life [19, 20]. This consequently leads to higher solid feed intake, greater BW gain, and easier transition from milk or milk replacer to diets based on solid feeds only. Therefore, grain based starter feeds are a standard part of diets for preweaned dairy calves.

Because some earlier studies showed that forage intake may even decrease intake of grain based starter by calves [21, 22], it has been a common recommendation to avoid feeding forages to calves, in order to prevent the delay of rumen development [1, 4]. In some countries, such as the US, such a recommendation is widespread by extension agents and online publications articles, such as that published by the Bovine Alliance on Management and Nutrition (BAMN) which is composed of representatives from American Association of Bovine Practitioners (AABP), American Dairy Science Association (ADSA), American Feed Industry Association (AFIA), and US Department of Agriculture (USDA) [5]. However, as forage supplementation research is continued, it has become recognized that forage intake for preweaned dairy calves is also important for rumen development. In nature, ruminants evolved to efficiently use forages and thus forage intake by newborn calves is what naturally would occur.

Forage intake stimulates rumen muscle growth and the development of rumination. Calves that were offered dry forages (grass hay, Lucerne hay or straw), in addition to grain sources, were shown to have greater rumen muscle thickness and rumination earlier in life, compared to calves that were fed only concentrates [7, 23, 24]. Furthermore, faster digesta passage out of the rumen was observed and many pathological changes within ruminal epithelium were reduced. Specifically, feeding solely grain based starter feed to calves oftentimes leads to para- and hyperkeratosis, which are evident by the formation of feed and hair plaques firmly attached to the rumen mucosa and ruminal epithelium para- and hyperkeratosis [25–27]. Forage particles present in the rumen stimulate rumen motility thereby preventing plaque formation [26, 27]; whereas, abrasiveness of forage particles enhances keratinized ruminal epithelial cell desquamation thereby preventing para- and hyperkeratosis [25, 28]. Simultaneously, increased rumen motility and digesta passage out of the rumen, in combination with increased time spent ruminating, prevents excessive ruminal pH drop, via increased volatile fatty acid (VFA) passage to the omasum and increased delivery of buffers to the rumen within saliva. A very low pH is commonly reported in calves fed grain based starter feeds ad libitum and there are indications that it may have a negative impact on performance of calves [29]. Beneficial impacts of forage intake on rumen development are further supported by higher expression of some VFA transporters in ruminal epithelium of calves offered forages in addition to grain based starter feed, compared to those fed only concentrates [7], indicating that the development of ruminal epithelium may also be, to some extent, positively affected by forage intake. When forages are offered, e.g. bulky feed, this also stimulates the development of rumen capacity [7, 19], which is very limited in calves in the first several weeks of life [30].

Altogether, forage intake stabilizes the rumen environment, affects rumen capacity development, and prevents rumen epithelium abnormalities. These positive impacts of forage intake by calves were accompanied by increased solid feed intake and ADG of calves in numerous studies (for details, see latter part of the chapter) [1–3]. Likely, forage feeding to preweaned dairy calves also prepares the rumen for efficient forage digestion after weaning; however, evidence of this is limited [1].

Besides beneficial impacts on rumen development, access to forage limits abnormal behavior of calves, [6, 24, 31, 32]. These behaviors, such as sucking, licking or biting different objects, other calves or themselves, are quite often reported in dairy calves that are kept individually and fed limited amounts of liquid feeds with access to grain based starter feed only. Thus, feeding forage to calves also should be considered from a welfare viewpoint.

3. How are dry and ensiled forages different, especially with regard to preweaned dairy calves?

3.1 Cost and labor

In 2015, an invited review described changes in the dairy industry in North America, Europe, Australia, and New Zealand. One important highlight was the low average number of cows per herd, which was largest in New Zealand, at over 400, and smallest in Norway and Germany, at under 50 [33]. Although only certain nations were reported, other developed and developing countries would most likely be similar, indicating that no matter the dairy cow population in the country, most dairy farms are still small in size. This is an important distinguishing feature of the dairy industry because smaller farms have less resources, labor, and equipment.

A feeding recommendation of adding forage to calf diets can come with unforeseen problems. If a small farm were to consider this recommendation, they would have to evaluate not only what forage to provide their calves but how to process this forage, which would add required labor and equipment use.

The availability of dried forages on a dairy farm varies. Many lactating rations use either straw to add roughage to the lactating diet or high quality hay for high producing animals. Even in areas of the world where dairy farms include a significant portion of hay in their ration, current farm data from the Midwest shows a reduction in hay fed to dairy cows. One of the reasons for this is due to the lack of available hay. Many areas in the US have a severely low hay inventory due to poor growing and drying conditions making this a feedstuff that is either unavailable or too costly [34].

The cost of good quality hay at 150 Relative Feed Quality (RFQ) can be priced up to 50% more than 100 RFQ hay [35]. Due to calves and heifers not providing a current income source, farmers may be hesitant to use a higher quality, more expensive hay to meet calf forage feeding recommendations. But using lower quality forages, with higher neutral detergent fiber (NDF) and lower RFQ, for feeding young calves can be detrimental to their growth and development. Specifically, when dry forages are used in calf diets not only as a supplement aiming to ensure 'optimal' rumen development and preventing stereotypic behavior, but also as an important source of nutrients, such as protein, low quality hay can significantly reduce nutrient intake [27, 36]. The cost and availability of higher quality forages may leave farmers little choice as to what to supplement their calf diets.

There are many ways to estimate the price of ensiled feeds; however, the result is always significantly less than dried forages. In the US, corn silage (CS) can be priced around $30 per ton, resulting in less than two pennies per pound of forage. Contrastingly, AH can cost around 10 cents per pound, depending on the RFQ and year of harvest. Additional time and labor also need to be taken into account since ensiled feeds are already chopped at the time of supplementation but dry forages need to be further chopped to provide calves with manageable (and also desirable, based on some studies; see latter parts of the chapter) particle length. Thus, feeding silages may be more justified than feeding dry forages due to lower costs, practical convenience, and higher accessibility on farms.

3.2 Moisture

The main difference between dry forages, such as hay and straw, and silages is moisture content, which is much higher for silages. The moisture of a feed can influence its palatability and acceptance for young dairy calves.

Kargar et al. [37, 38] fed reconstituted hay soaked in water to a dry matter (DM) content of 20%. When dry hay was replaced in the same concentrations in the calf starter with the moist hay, calves had similar DM intake (DMI) and ADG but digestibility of NDF was higher, and fecal scores and general appearance were also better as moisture increased. Similarly, Beiranvand et al. [39, 40] added water directly to starter diets in the summer and winter. They found that increasing moisture levels from 10 to 50% linearly increased DMI, ADG, and rumen VFA production, compared to calves eating dry calf starter in hot weather. Thus, adding a moist forage source, such as a silage, would not only provide necessary fiber to stabilize the developing rumen environment but may enhance feed intake by reducing dustiness and increasing palatability of dry, fine or pelleted calf starters.

Although soaking dry forages is difficult to apply on farm, adding water to calf starter that is already mixed with processed dry forages (e.g. chopped hay) is a possible method to enhancing starter intake. However, practical applications are also limited, especially in cold weather where water would freeze. Hot weather may also cause practical handling issues where higher moisture feeds can heat up. Although water soaked calf starter may have this problem, silage would also be difficult to handle during hot temperatures. Felton and DeVries [41] added water to a TMR for lactating cows and found an increase in feed temperature by the end of the day due to microbial respiration. This may reduce feed intake since hot silage is indicative of feed spoilage. Therefore, if silages are provided to calves, they must be changed out daily so as to prevent any palatability issues.

3.3 Forage particle length and processing

As already mentioned, the preweaned calf rumen is small and underdeveloped with a lower digestive capability and capacity. During calf growth and development, rumen weight (both full and empty) expressed as a proportion of BW increases up to the age of six months, indicating its immaturity within this period of life [30]. This immaturity especially limits intake of voluminous feeds, such as forages. This, in turn, requires solid feedstuffs provided to calves to be less bulky and more digestible as calf rumens fill quickly with less digestible feeds.

Dry forages can be fed to calves without processing or being processed prior to feeding, e.g. chopped to reduce their bulkiness to make feeding and prehension easier. Nevertheless, when calves were fed long or chopped hay, the former one was more willingly consumed, indicating that calves prefer long dry forages [42]. There are also indications that long, dry forages may be more effective in preventing stereotypic behavior of young calves [43]. However, intake of long hay was shown to vary substantially between calves and results in a lot of waste where hay is removed from hay racks but not eaten [44]. Furthermore, because intake of long hay by some animals may account for 20% of consumed DM this may reduce intake of concentrates, efficiency of nutrient digestion, and growth of calves preweaning, as shown in several studies [31, 36, 45]. Therefore, if dry forages are fed to calves, such as hay or straw, they should be fed chopped (e.g. 2–4 cm long) and offered limited amounts in order to prevent feed waste and performance reduction due to higher intakes of feed that is not easily digested. However, chopping of dry forages requires more efforts, labor, and costs associated with feeding calves. Particularly, suitable equipment for chopping dry forages may be a limitation for some farms.

Ensiled forages are typically chopped before fermentation which reduces the bulkiness of the feedstuff. For example, CS is harvested and chopped to primarily provide adequate physically effective NDF (peNDF) to lactating dairy cows. Although variable from farm to farm and dependent on many factors, theoretical length of cut (TLC) of CS averages $^{3/8}$ – ¾ of an inch and geometric mean averages 9.5 mm [45]. The threshold particle size of particles leaving the rumen in adult cattle was reported to be under 1.18 mm geometric mean [46]. With an average geometric mean of 9.5 mm, chopped CS will increase rumen fill, however, not to the extent of long-stemmed hay; this average length should also stimulate chewing to help regulate rumen pH. Actually, there are reports indicating that providing chopped CS to calves affects rumination and feeding behavior [6, 43]. Using a chopped forage source compared with simply providing long-stemmed hay or straw will reduce rumen fill and allow the calf to eat more starter grain. Many farms also utilize an additional step prior to ensiling to further 'destroy' structure of the plant material and thus increase its digestibility in the rumen. This applies especially for whole plant CS by using processing rolls which reduce particle size and increase starch digestibility for better silage fermentation [47]. This allows the protein matrix that encapsulates the starch to be disrupted thereby improving fermentation. For a pre-ruminant with low rumen digestibility, these chopping and processing methods can allow easier utilization of nutrients. Research feeding different processed corn types within a texturized starter to calves reported the type of processed corn can influence intake, growth, and rumen parameters [48]. Various parameters were affected differently depending on whether calves received whole, roasted rolled, dry rolled or steam flaked corn within their texturized starter. Not one of these corn types was overall better than another but if ensiled feeds are processed, this may affect calf performance.

Nevertheless, the optimal particle size of forage may differ depending on inclusion of forages in the diet. Results from research using short AH at 2.92 mm compared to long at 5.04 mm (as geometric means) with low inclusion at 8% and high inclusion at 16%, on a DM basis in starter feed, showed that particle size may inhibit calf performance. If calves were fed the longer particle size, they did best with the lower inclusion level. And calves that were fed shorter particle size did best with the higher inclusion level, indicating there is a balance between length and volume of forage included in calf diets [36].

It has to be also mentioned, that forages that are finely chopped or pelleted have no beneficial impact on rumen function or performance of calves [48].

3.4 Forage type and its nutritional value

Various plant materials can be dried or ensiled, resulting in different hays and silages. The nutritive value, particularly digestibility, may differ, affecting performance of animals. For example, when grass from the same sward was dried or ensiled, NDF digestibility was higher for resulting hay than silage in bulls [49, 50]. However, studies comparing feeding the same plant material dried or ensiled to calves on nutrient digestibility and their performance are lacking. Thus, an unequivocal answer to the question of whether dried or ensiled forage is a better source of nutrients for preweaned calves cannot be given.

Nevertheless, when it comes to dried forages, studies indicate that those having higher nutritive value (e.g. higher crude protein (CP) and lower fiber concentration), such as good quality grass or AH, are more willingly consumed by calves than those having lower nutritive value, such as straw [6]. However, good quality grass hay or AH feeding to calves was shown to reduce intake of grain based starter feed and feed efficiency, thus negatively affecting growth of calves and costs of rearing [3, 6, 43]. Therefore, feeding chopped straw to calves may be an even better option than feeding chopped grass hay or AH. Such an option may be especially attractive for farms that contend with limited resources of good quality hay. When straw is used in diets for calves, the aim of its feeding is simply to include forage in the diet in order to ensure proper physical stimulation for the rumen, rumination, and to limit stereotypic behavior of animals.

On the other hand, not many studies compare impact of various ensiled forages on feed intake and performance of calves. Of those available, triticale silage was more willingly consumed by calves than CS, and also its feeding resulted in higher starter feed intake; however, ADG of calves and FE was not affected [6]. Nevertheless, in the majority of studies, CS feeding to calves was investigated (see **Table 1**) due to common usage of this feed in dairy production. Compared to other forages, CS has also substantial starch content. Thus, this feed can be considered as not only a source of fiber and physical structure in the diet, but also a source of easily fermentable starch in the rumen. Whole crop silages may, therefore, be an especially attractive source of forage for preweaned calves.

3.5 Microbials

The principle of silage fermentation is to convert water-soluble carbohydrates into organic acids. In an anaerobic environment, lactic acid bacteria are able to rapidly reduce the pH and increase stability of the silage. The resulting fermented product contains populations of lactobacilli and other microbial species [56] that, in general, are lacking in dry forages.

There have been hundreds of published papers evaluating probiotics and their effects on health and productive parameters of dairy calves. From meta-analyses, many reviews present nonsignificant or positive responses in growth, feed efficiency, and health when microbial-based products have been fed to growing calves [57]. Conclusions tend to support the use of probiotics as low risk with a potential positive benefit for the growing calf.

Many of these probiotics include lactobacilli species which are also found in properly fermented silages. Hypothetically, the question would be whether supplementing calves with silage could potentially enhance their rumen and intestinal microbiota similar to probiotic supplements available on the market. Xu et al. [58] evaluated the use of *Saccharomyces cerevisiae*, which is reported to promote rumen development, as a silage inoculant. In the fermented silage end product, they found higher microbial communities of *S. cerevisiae*, which further increased in abundance after aerobic exposure. Furthermore, one study reported positive effects feeding *Lactobacillus plantarum*, a commonly used silage inoculant, to preweaned dairy calves. The treatments of *L. plantarum* were fed to calves at 0, 4, and 8 g/day resulting in positive linear growth and fecal score improvements [59]. Other research is being conducted to determine whether some of these silage inoculant bacteria types may help enhance the health and performance of animals when directly fed. This could also be an added benefit for supplementing growing dairy calves with ensiled feeds.

Forage source[1]	Calves/ trmt	Start (d)	Weaning (d)	Forage (%)	Feeding method[2]	Starter form	ADG	DMI	FE[3]	Rumen[4]	Reference
Sta + AH, Sta + CS, Sta + AH + CS	10	3	50	10, 10, 5	TMR	Fine ground	NS	NS	ND	ND	Kargar et al. [37]
Sta + CS, Sta + RAH Sta + RBP	18	3	50	10	TMR	Ground	NS[5]	NS	NS	NS	Kargar et al. [38]
Sta, Sta + CS, CS	15	3	49	0, 50, 100	TMR	Texturized	NS	NS	NS	- CS	Kehoe et al. [51]
Sta, Sta + AH, Sta + CS	10	3	49	0, 15, 15	TMR	Fine ground	+ CS	+ CS	ND[6]	+ CS	Mirzaei et al. [32]
Sta, Sta + CS	12	3	56	0, 15	TMR	Ground, pelleted	+ CS	NS	NS	+pH, +acetate	Mirzaei et al. [52]
Sta, Sta + GH TMR, Sta + GH sep, TMR	6	1	50	0, 15, Ad lib, 71	Variable	Texturized	NS	- TMR	NS	NS	Overvest et al. [53]
Sta, TS, CS	20	14.1 +/− 4.2	57	Ad libitum	Free choice	Pelleted	+ TS, CS	+ TS	NS	ND	Castells et al. [6]
Sta, Sta + CS	8	10	70	0, 30, 60	TMR	Pelleted	NS	NS	NS	- CS	Suarez et al. [54]
Sta + CS	10	8	35	0, 33.7	TMR	Ground	NS	NS	ND	+ CS	Block and Shellenberger [55]

[1]*Sta: Calf starter treatment without forage inclusion, RAH: Reconstituted alfalfa hay; RBP: reconstituted beet pulp, AH: Alfalfa hay, CS: corn silage, GH: grass hay, Sta + GH sep: Starter and grass hay fed separately.*
[2]*TMR: Total mixed ration based on 37% CS and 34% legume haylage, TS: Triticale silage.*
[3]*FE: Gain to feed ratio.*
[4]*Rumen: Rumen development parameters evaluated by BHB concentrations, pH, VFAs or physical appearance including papillae parameters.*
[5]*NS: Not significant ($P \geq 0.05$).*
[6]*ND: Not determined.*

Table 1.
A summary of studies evaluating corn silage in pre-weaned dairy calf diets.

3.6 Palatability

Palatability is defined as the collective aspects of a feed material that are sensed before being swallowed. Adult cows have been reported to enjoy sweet and umami flavors and avoid bitter tastes although not to the extent as other mammals, such as sheep [60]. There are few research studies that report on palatability in calves. Calf palatability and preference have been researched mostly in regard to ingredient use in calf starters. Calves have clear preferences for certain ingredients that should be considered when formulating their feedstuffs. Wheat meal and soybean meal were most preferred; however, previous experience with these ingredients, difference in age, and current nutrition status (whether receiving enough milk and nutrients) can play an influential role [61]. On the other hand, no typical preference tests for forages were conducted in calves. However, based on results of Castells et al. [6] it can be concluded that AH and oat hay is more willingly consumed by preweaned calves, and thus likely more palatable, than ryegrass hay, barley straw, CS, and triticale silage.

As opposed to dry forages, silages are acidic and this acidic taste may potentially affect their intake. Similar to what is known for adult cattle, calves have a preference for sweet flavors such as found in whole milk [62]. However, they will consume feedstuffs with a lower pH, such as acidified milk and milk replacer, which have been fed for decades to preweaned dairy calves. In the US, 1.7% of farms feed acidified milk by using an organic acid to preserve the milk so it can be stored and fed at ambient temperatures [63]. Typical pH range of acidified milk or milk replacer can be anywhere from 5.5 to as low as 4.0; if pH drops too low, research has found decreased intake as reported with acidification with citric acid between a pH of 4.2 and 5.2 [64]. Since silages can be acidified anywhere from 3.8–5.5 depending on their forage source [56], it can be speculated that this may have some inhibitory effect on palatability and DMI. Nevertheless, studies conducted so far indicate that at least palatability of CS or triticale silage for calves is more or less comparable to palatability of different dry forages [6, 32].

It is also worth mentioning that the preference for certain tastes can result from the nutrients contained in the feedstuff. For example, sweet flavor may be preferred due the correlation with the presence of carbohydrates and umami may be preferred due to the presence of amino acids within the feedstuff. In adult animals, post-ingestive feedback plays a large role in preference for feed types [65]; however, preweaned calves have a low solid feed intake and may not be influenced by this.

4. What are the effects of feeding silage on performance parameters in dairy calves?

Taking into account information presented in previous paragraphs, silages possess potential advantages and disadvantages when it comes to feeding them to preweaned calves. Hence, the following paragraphs will focus on the effects of feeding ensiled feedstuffs on rumen development and digestibility, feed intake, and growth and health parameters in preweaned dairy calves and will discuss those in terms of practical application of silages in calf diets.

4.1 Rumen development and digestibility

The impact of forage quality and quantity has been well established in lactating cows and has also been shown in previous reviews to affect preweaned calves [2, 3]. In this review, which focuses solely on silages, there seems to be a similar impact on rumen development and rumen functions of feeding silage in addition to calf starter as dry forages, compared to feeding calf starter only.

When CS was provided to calves in addition to calf starter, rumen pH significantly increased compared to only calf starter feeding [32, 52]. This ensiled forage source acts similarly to its inclusion in lactating rations, stimulating chewing to increase saliva and buffer the VFAs and resulting acids in the rumen. Calves that are fed a readily fermentable feed, such as a ground or fine calf starter can develop low rumen pH which can lead to keratinization and ulceration of the rumen wall and feed plaque formation [25, 27, 66]. At day 35, calves fed CS mixed with ground or texturized starter had higher ruminal pH (5.98 vs. 5.31) compared to calves that did not receive CS in their starter [52]. Calves that were fed AH, CS or a mixture of both, tended to increase their meal length and decrease their eating rate when fed CS compared with AH but significantly increased their rumination length [67]. This indicates that although CS did not take as long to eat as AH, calves spent time ruminating which would lead to increased salivation and improved rumen environment via delivery of more buffering substances into the rumen.

High fiber and high DMI diets tend to decrease digestibility in weaned calves [68, 69] so it is important to evaluate whether the addition of a forage source would reduce feedstuff digestibility in the preweaned calf. Adding forage to preweaned calf diets increases the fiber content of the diet which may lead to a decrease in digestibility and nutrient intake. Calves that were supplemented with triticale silage had greater CP intake compared to control calves fed only calf starter (235 vs. 171 g/d) but due to the higher fiber and bulkiness of the triticale silage, CP content of the total diet consumed relative to the control calves was actually decreased by 0.4 percentage units. However, an increase was seen in CP digestibility when calves were offered (in addition to starter feed) AH, rye hay, and CS compared to control, oat hay and barley straw with triticale silage being intermediate [6]. The digestibility of NDF in CS treatment was also significantly higher than AH soaked in water [38] which may be attributed to the fermentation the corn plant undergoes in the silo [70]. This is a positive effect since the microbes have begun the process of breaking down the nutrients thereby making it easier for the pre-ruminant calf to access them in their underdeveloped rumen environment. Although the bulkiness of silages can reduce the total intake of nutrients, because the digestibility of these nutrients increases, there is no negative impact on calf performance, especially when silage is fed in addition to starter feed, since the overall amount fed is rather small [6].

The evaluation of rumen parameters from the previous section, and also from other research trials, include physical rumen appearance of color and feed plaque formation, rumen papillae morphology, rumen papillae density, and rumen wall thickness. In studies conducted in 1980, calves fed CS had significantly shorter papillae (0.9, 3.5, 1.6 cm^3 for CS, pellets, and wood fines, respectively) but those were more dense (118.1, 51.9, 66.4 No./cm^2 for CS, pellets, and wood fines, respectively) compared to calves fed pellets or pellets with wood fines [55]. In a different study, 100% of calves fed solely calf starter had rumen plaque compared with 63% of calves fed a mixture of 40:60 starter and CS and 88% of calves fed 70:30 starter and CS. Additionally, 25% of calves fed 40:60 mixture had poor development of mucosa [54]. Rumen weight was highest and ventral muscle thickness was lowest for calves fed calf starter only compared to treatments receiving CS. The authors hypothesized that this may be influenced by feed plaque formation. Although the plaque formation was concerning, the authors concluded that microscopic evaluation of the rumen was not significantly different among treatments and that, overall, calves were healthy and silage can be added to the diet [54].

In a study in which calves were fed solely with CS without calf starter, reduced papillae length and width was observed, compared with calves fed CS and starter

(50:50 DM) and calves fed only calf starter. Papillae concentration was not different from the CS and starter mixture with CS but denser than calf starter alone [51]. Only this study evaluated intestinal morphology where CS treatment had the shortest crypt depth and mucosa thickness (villus length plus crypt depth). The authors hypothesized that lower dietary protein intake in CS only calves could have been one of the factors leading to these results; a lack of calf starter in the diet would not only reduce VFA production but dietary protein intake since CS is low in CP. This morphology indicates a potential reduction of surface area for nutrient absorption in the rumen as well as epithelial cell proliferation in the intestine.

Butyrate concentration in the rumen has long been a standard indicator of the potential of a feed to stimulate rumen development in the calf because it is the main stimulatory VFA for rumen epithelial development [71]. It should follow that the metabolized form of butyrate, ß-hydroxybutyrate (BHB), should be increased in the blood if feed consumed promotes ruminal butyrate production, and thus enhances rumen development. In fact, the supplementation of sodium butyrate in the feed has been reported to improve rumen and gastrointestinal development in preweaned calves [72]. Although not all silage research trials reported on rumen development, of the ones that did, only a few showed increases in blood BHB or other rumen parameters when calves were fed silages. For example, calves fed CS were reported to have lower blood BHB concentrations [37], not different [51, 53] or higher BHB blood concentrations [32], compared to calves fed diets without silages. Therefore, blood BHB concentration may not be the best indicator of rumen development and potential of a feed to stimulate rumen development since it may be strongly influenced by differences in trial methods, such as starter quality, forage type, and forage quality or quantity.

The type of starter fed has an influence on how forage inclusion affects rumen parameters. When calves were fed a pelleted versus texturized starter with or without forage inclusion, calves receiving the pelleted starter with forage had a higher rumen fluid pH and intake than calves on just the pelleted starter. Similarly, calves receiving texturized starter had similar rumen pH to calves fed the pelleted starter with forage [9]. This indicates that forage is especially appropriate to include in the diet when the type of starter provided leads to apparent reduction in rumen pH. Adding a dry forage source to a pelleted starter has also been shown to increase post-weaning DMI and live weight [24, 73]. The only available study suggests that when ensiled feed (CS) is combined with a different form of starter feed, no impact on rumen pH can be expected; however, in that study, starter feed form (mesh or texturized) also had no impact on rumen pH [52]. Dry forage has different qualities from ensiled forage so more research needs to be done to discover whether a similar impact on rumen pH can be expected depending on the physical form of starter feed offered to calves. Also, different types of starter quality makes it difficult to compare results from research projects attempting to evaluate forage effectiveness in calf diets. However, the cost of pelleted or ground calf starter is lower than a texturized starter, making it more attractive to farms looking to reduce cost; forage supplementation may positively affect feeding such starter feeds or even may be required.

In summary, supplementing preweaned calves with ensiled feeds results in variable rumen development and nutrient digestibility. About half of the trials reported benefits and the other half reported reductions in either pH, VFAs or morphometric analyses.

4.2 Feed intake parameters

In older dairy cattle, particle length and moisture content can affect DMI but, as seen in **Table 1**, the majority of research trials evaluating feeding silages to calves compared to feeding dry forages or only calf starter reported no differences in DMI.

Only Castells et al. [6] did find lower intake of silages compared to some (but not all) dry forages tested in their study. However, in their study, calves were offered silages separately from starter feed, allowing them to choose to consume it rather than being 'force-fed' in a TMR protocol such as in other trials. This caused forage intake to decrease but inversely increased calf starter intake [6]. Although triticale silage and CS were consumed at only half the amount of AH and oat hays, similarly to rye hay and barley straw, the calves having access to silages increased starter consumption to a higher level than calves fed AH. In fact, triticale silage significantly increased total DMI and ADG compared to calves fed only starter and AH. This could be due to rumen fill [1]; however, considering intake of the triticale silage was only half of AH, this is not likely. Calves offered CS had greater ADG than calves fed only starter, although in the end, there were no differences between any treatments for gain to feed ratios. Thus, method of feeding ensiled forages may be an important factor affecting final results of their use in diets for calves. Perhaps the silage pH may inhibit its willing consumption, as discussed previously, or simply silages fed separately are more difficult to eat. Nevertheless, feeding ensiled forages as a mixture with grain based starter feed seems the best option to ensure ensiled forages are willingly consumed.

Mirzaei et al. [32] reported a significant increase of DMI when starter feed was mixed with CS compared to AH. The increase in dietary moisture level may have increased digestibility [37, 38], and thus feed intake, or palatability, by reducing dustiness of the TMR. Supportive of the latter, when calves were fed CS compared to reconstituted AH, where AH was soaked in water to reach a moisture of 20% DM to match the DM% of CS provided, no differences were reported in overall feed intake [37, 38]. This indicates that moisture may play a role in palatability and DMI of calves. Contrary to this, calves fed a TMR based on CS and legume haylage had significantly reduced DMI, although as-fed feed intake was not different from calves fed only starter, or starter supplemented with chopped grass hay in TMR or chopped grass hay separately. The TMR had significantly lower DM% at 51% compared with the other treatments which all were 88–90% concluding that calves were unable to eat enough DM to make up for the higher moisture [53].

Thus, keeping in mind calf palatability and digestive capacity, the amount of forage provided should be restricted if mixed in a TMR fashion. When calves were allowed to choose how much forage they ate with their calf starter, silages were consumed at 4 and 5% for triticale and corn silage, respectively [6]. Dried forages were not much higher at 8, 5, and 4% for oat hay, barley straw, and rye hay, respectively. Other research trials have fed a TMR style where percentages were anywhere from 30 to 60% of DM [51, 54] and some positive effects, such as increasing DMI, ADG or FE were not seen. It has been shown that mixing forages at higher levels (up to 10% DM) can reduce ADG and DMI [21, 22]. Based on result of studies in which ensiled forages were fed as a mixture with starter feed it seems that their inclusion of up to 15% of DM does not negatively affect DMI [32, 52].

Some of the lack of differences in DMI may relate to the type of calf starter fed with the forage, as already discussed for potential interaction between forage type and starter feed form. Corn silage mixed with a pelleted starter containing either barley grain or corn grain increased overall and post-weaning feed intake as compared to AH fed with either grain [32]. Others also found an increase in DMI with a pelleted starter [6]. On the other hand, different researchers that fed a texturized starter saw no differences in performance parameters for calves fed with or without CS [51, 52], although feed intake was increased in some of those when CS was mixed with texturized starter [52]. Another research study using a pelleted starter found an increase in CS DMI compared with a diet with added straw but no differences compared to the control treatment fed only calf starter [54]. More studies in dairy calves are needed on the form of starter feed and particle size of ensiled feeds and their effects on DMI.

In summary, feeding ensiled forages to calves has little effect on DMI and FE. The moisture difference of silage compared to dry forages or only calf starter may increase palatability of feed for preweaned dairy calves. However, more research is needed on the interaction of starter feed form and particle size of ensiled feeds. Keeping silage inclusion below 15% of DM is important to allow for calves to intake their solid feed to their full potential.

4.3 Growth and health parameters

The increase of DMI will usually increase BW and ADG due to an increase in nutrient intake. Because in the majority of studies in which ensiled forages were fed to calves, overall DMI was increased (**Table 1**), BW and ADG of animals were also positively affected. For example, regardless of calf starter form (mash vs. textured), calves receiving CS had significantly greater preweaning ADG (564 vs. 411 g/d) and overall ADG (598 vs. 443 g/d; 61) compared to calves not receiving CS in their diet.

An obvious explanation for this is already discussed and reported in numerous studies explaining the positive impact of feeding forages on rumen environment, nutrient digestibility, or both. Another explanation, already partially discussed, could be that ensiled feeds, especially CS, contain higher levels of digestible starch which is a valuable nutrient addition to the rumen environment. Since most trials discussed in this paper utilize CS as the main ensiled feed, it is important to keep in mind that other ensiled feeds may have different results. Starch content and digestibility in CS is much higher than in hays such as AH and, especially, straw. The starch content of CS is typically 25 to 35% and starch digestibility of CS that has been kernel processed can be over 87%. In comparison to AH and straw, which contain mostly structural carbohydrates and little starch [74], CS starch content can improve the rumen environment. And lastly, a third explanation could be that calves receiving forage ruminated more and had reduced nonnutritive behaviors, which would lead to greater DMI and, therefore, ADG [6, 32]. Interestingly, these two research trials found opposite effects where Mirzaei et al. [32] reported calves supplemented with CS spent more time ruminating compared with AH but Castells et al. [6] reported calves fed AH spent more time ruminating compared to other groups, including the CS group. The difference may be with the feeding method where the former trial fed a TMR and the latter trial fed starter and forage separately. However, both trials found that non-forage supplemented treatments had the lowest rumination times and highest non-nutritive oral behaviors as well as lower feed intake and ADG.

Other studies evaluating ensiled forage compared with a dry hay or only calf starter reported no differences in BW or nutrient intake. Research using veal calves concluded that forage may be added to the veal calf diet since performance parameters were not affected. No difference in BW at slaughter was reported with ADG ranging from 688 to 779 g/d [54]. Even in research where DMI was reduced in calves fed TMR (a silage based lactating ration TMR) with a low DM (51.5% DM), due to higher milk intakes, calves were able to maintain their ADG until weaning [53]. Once at weaning and during post-weaning, TMR fed calves reduced ADG due to the higher moisture content and diluted nutrient content compared with calves receiving starter, starter mixed with grass hay, and starter fed separately from grass hay.

Health scores of calves, if reported, were also not different for most trials [38, 51, 52]. One research trial reported a tendency of higher rectal temperature probability (≥40°C) before weaning in CS fed calves compared to calves fed reconstituted beet pulp, which was soaked in water to 20% DM ($P \leq 0.08$) and a lower probability of having pneumonia ($P \leq 0.09$). Since number of days and treatment frequency were not different, it was concluded that calves were in general very healthy and these data were unusual [38]. Overall, the addition of ensiled forages to calf diets has no effect on health parameters.

In summary, although there were some negative rumen parameter and digestibility effects, ensiled feeds either had no effect or a positive effect on other performance parameters, such as ADG and health. If a farmer were to incorporate ensiled feeds into their calf nutrition plan, they would most likely see positive or no effects on calf growth, health and feed intake.

5. Potential limitations of feeding ensiled forages to calves

As with any new practical application, the addition of ensiled forages to calf diets needs to be evaluated carefully on each farm. There are limitations that come with the addition of ensiled forages to calf diets. But with careful management, these can be overcome and this type of feedstuff can become useful and advantageous for use on farm.

As mentioned in a previous section, ensiled feed will heat up during the day when exposed to oxygen. This indicates bacterial respiration which can not only reduce nutrients and DM but palatability [75]. Because silages are made throughout the world, there are challenges to overcome when ensiling forages, especially in hot or cold climates [76]. Although most of the studies reviewed in this chapter have not found reductions in silage consumption if fed in low amounts in TMR style, feeding well fermented silage needs to be a priority; young animals are typically most susceptible to poor nutrition.

With increasing knowledge of proper ensiling practices, it is well known that mycotoxins may be produced when silage is not properly fermented [77]. Mycotoxins are secondary metabolites of fungi that may be produced due to a number of different factors, such as weather, improper packing and sealing, and forage quality and moisture. They can cause adverse health effects and have been reported in young growing animals, such as juvenile goats, to reduce growth and immune system function [78]. When considering the addition of ensiled feeds to calf diets, the quality of the ensiled feed needs to be evaluated. Spoiled or hot silage should not be fed to young animals.

Although this chapter refers to silages in general, most research has been done with CS. Only one of the research papers presented used triticale silage with all others using CS [6]. The nutritional properties of CS compared to other silages being used worldwide, such as oatlage, barlage, or sugar cane silage, can be very different in nutritional content. It is important to keep this in mind when considering the implementation of feeding ensiled forage to calves.

All of these limitations can be overcome with careful management and planning. To overcome these limitations, farmers should consider their calf feeding management. If the farm is able to change out solid feed on a daily basis, the old, heated silage will be replaced with more palatable feed. If the farm is currently using proper silage management techniques during harvesting, storage, and feedout, this will reduce the chances of mycotoxins being fed to young calves. And if the farm feeds a different silage than CS, they should consider its slow incorporation and evaluating its effects on their calves since more research needs to be done using different ensiled forages in calf diets.

6. Conclusions

Corn silage (CS), haylage, and other small grain and grass silages are fermented to improve digestibility and nutrient access which can be beneficial to animals whose rumen is not fully developed. Silages also contain other byproducts such as active microbes that may be beneficial in a probiotic sense. With the reduced accessibility of good quality hay in certain parts of the world, silages may be the answer as a common feedstuff found on farm that is low in cost for the farmer. Without the need of further processing, silages can be easily utilized in a preweaned calf diet.

As dairy markets continue to be volatile and farmers are faced with tough economic choices, the search continues for providing good quality feed at a lower cost. Research shows that the addition of silage to calf feed either does not affect or may have a positive influence on calf growth and performance. Although some trials reported some reduction in rumen parameters, at the same time these trials showed no differences in calf growth and health compared to no forage or other forage treatments. Keeping in mind some limitations of ensiled forages, this review indicates that silages may be used for preweaned calf diets. Silage management is important since this fermented feed may heat during the day; using small amounts mixed into calf starter like a TMR and providing fresh silage daily can allow ensiled feeds to be easily incorporated into calf diets on farm. Further research is required with different types of silages and mixtures and each farmer should assess this available feedstuff carefully on their own farm.

Author details

Sylvia I. Kehoe[1]*, Paweł Górka[2] and Zhijun J. Cao[3]

1 University of Wisconsin-River Falls, River Falls, USA

2 University of Agriculture in Krakow, Krakow, Poland

3 China Agricultural University, Beijing, China

*Address all correspondence to: sylvia.kehoe@uwrf.edu

References

[1] Khan MA, Bach A, Weary DM, von Keyserlingk MAG: Invited review: Transitioning from milk to solid feed in dairy heifers. J Dairy Sci. 2016;99:885-902. DOI: 10.3168/jds.2015-9975

[2] Xiao J, Alugongo GM, Li J, Wang Y, Li S, Cao Z: Review: How forage feeding early in life influences the growth rate, ruminal environment, and the establishment of feeding behavior in pre-weaned calves. Animals (Basel). 2020;10:188. DOI: 10.3390/ANI10020188

[3] Imani M, Mirzaei M, Baghbanzadeh-Nobari B, Ghaffari MH: Effects of forage provision to dairy calves on growth performance and rumen fermentation: A meta-analysis and meta-regression. J Dairy Sci. 2017;100:1136-1150. DOI: 10.3168/jds.2016-11561.

[4] Heinrichs AJ: Rumen development in the dairy calf. Adv Dairy Tech. 2005;17: 179-187

[5] BAMN: A guide to feeding and weaning healthy and productive dairy calves. 2017. AFIA Publications. Available from: https://www.aphis.usda.gov/animal_health/nahms/dairy/downloads/bamn/BAMN17_GuideFeeding_1.pdf. [Accessed: 2021-05-05].

[6] Castells L, Bach A, Araujo G, Montoro C, Terré M: Effect of different forage sources on performance and feeding behavior of Holstein calves. J Dairy Sci. 2012;95:286-293. DOI: 10.3168/JDS.2011-4405

[7] Castells L, Bach A, Aris A, Terré M: Effects of forage provision to young calves on rumen fermentation and development of the gastrointestinal tract. J Dairy Sci. 2013;96:5226-5236. DOI: 10.3168/jds.2012-6419

[8] Kowalski ZM, Gorka P, Schlagheck A, Jagusiak W, Micek P, Strzetelski J: Performance of Holstein calves fed milk-replacer and starter mixture supplemented with probiotic feed additive. J Anim Feed Sci. 2009;18:399-411. DOI: 10.22358/jafs/66409/2009

[9] Terré M, Castells L, Khan MA, Bach A: Interaction between the physical form of the starter feed and straw provision on growth performance of Holstein calves. J Dairy Sci. 2015;98:1101-1109. DOI: 10.3168/JDS.2014-8151

[10] Strzetelski JA, Brzóska F, Kowalski ZM, Osięgłowski S: Feeding recommendation for Ruminants and Feed Tables. Fundacja Insytytutu Zootechniki PIB, Propanus Animalium, Kraków (in Polish). 2014.

[11] Johnson KF, Chancellor N, Burn CC, Wathes DC: Analysis of pre-weaning feeding policies and other risk factors influencing growth rates in calves on 11 commercial dairy farms. Animal. 2017;12:1413-1423. DOI: 10.1017/S1751731117003160

[12] Medrano-Galarza C, LeBlanc SJ, DeVries TJ, Jones-Bitton A, Rushen J, de Passillé AM, Haley DB: A survey of dairy calf management practices among farms using manual and automated milk feeding systems in Canada. J Dairy Sci. 2017;100:6872-6884. DOI: 10.3168/JDS.2016-12273

[13] Phipps A, Beggs D, Murray A, Mansell P, Pyman M: A survey of northern Victorian dairy farmers to investigate dairy calf management: calf-rearing practices. Australian Vet J. 2018;96:107-110. DOI: 10.1111/AVJ.12686

[14] Flaga J, Górka P, Kowalski ZM, Kaczor U, Pietrzak P, Zabielski R: Insulin-like growth factors 1 and 2 (IGF-1 and IGF-2) mRNA levels in relation to the gastrointestinal tract (GIT) development in newborn calves.

Pol J Vet Sci. 2011;14:605-613. DOI: 10.2478/v10181-011-0090-z

[15] Stabo IJF, Joy JHB, Gaston HJ: Rumen development in the calf: 2. The effect of diets containing different proportion of concentrates to hay on digestive efficiency. British J Nutr. 1966;20:189-215. DOI: 10.1079/bjn19660022

[16] Bergman EN: Energy contributions of volatile fatty acids from the gastrointestinal tract in various species. Physiol Rev. 1990;70:567-590. DOI: 10.1152/physrev.1990.70.2.567

[17] Mentschel J, Leiser R, Mülling C, Pfarrer C, Claus R: Butyric acid stimulates rumen mucosa development in the calf mainly by a reduction of apoptosis. Arch Tierernahr. 2001;55:85-102. DOI: 10.1080/17450390109386185

[18] Malhi M, Gui H, Yao L, Aschenbach JR, Gabel G, and Shen Z: Increased papillae growth and enhanced short-chain fatty acid absorption in the rumen of goats are associated with transient increases in cyclin D1 expression after ruminal butyrate infusion. J Dairy Sci. 2013;96:7603-7616. DOI: 10.3168/jds.2013-6700

[19] Tamate H, McGilliard AD, Jacobson NL, Getty R: Effect of various dietaries on the anatomical development of the stomach in the calf. J. Dairy Sci. 1962;45:408-420. DOI:10.3168/JDS.S0022-0302(62)89406-5

[20] Connor EE, Baldwin 6th RL, Li CJ, Li RW, Chung H: Gene expression in bovine rumen epithelium during weaning identifies molecular regulators of rumen development and growth. Funct Integr Genomics. 2013;13:133-142. DOI: 10.1007/s10142-012-0308-x

[21] Hill TM, Bateman HG, Aldrich JM, Schlotterbeck RL: Effects of the amount of chopped hay or cottonseed hulls in a textured calf starter on young calf performance. J Dairy Sci. 2008;91:2684-2693. DOI: 10.3168/JDS.2007-0935

[22] Hill TM, Bateman HG, Aldrich JM, Schlotterbeck RL: Roughage amount, source, and processing for diets fed to weaned dairy calves. Prof Anim Sci. 2010;26:181-187. DOI: 10.15232/S1080-7446(15)30578-7

[23] Nocek JE, Heald CW, Polan CE: Influence of ration physical form and nitrogen availability on ruminal morphology of growing bull calves. J Dairy Sci. 1984;67:334-343. DOI: 10.3168/jds.S0022-0302(84)81306-5

[24] Terré M, Pedrals E, Dalmau A, Bach A: What do preweaned and weaned calves need in the diet: a high fiber content or a forage source? J Dairy Sci. 2013;96:5217-5225. DOI: 10.3168/JDS.2012-6304

[25] Beharka AA, Nagaraja TG, Morrill JL, Kennedy GA, Klemm RD: Effects of form of the diet on anatomical, microbial, and fermentative development of the rumen of neonatal calves. J Dairy Sci. 1998;81: 1946-1955. DOI: 10.3168/jds.S0022-0302(98)75768-6

[26] Suárez BJ, Reenen CGV, Stockhofe N, Dijkstra J, Gerrits WJJ: Effect of roughage source and roughage to concentrate ratio on animal performance and rumen development in veal calves. J Dairy Sci. 2007;90:2390-2403. DOI: 10.3168/JDS.2006-524

[27] Pazoki A, Ghorbani GR, Kargar S, Sadeghi-Sefidmazgi A, Drackley JK, Ghaffari MH: Growth performance, nutrient digestibility, ruminal fermentation, and rumen development of calves during transition from liquid to solid feed: Effects of physical form of starter feed and forage provision. Anim Feed Sci Technol. 2017;234:173-185. DOI: 10.1016/j.anifeedsci.2017.06.004

[28] Greenwood RH, Morrill JL, Titgemeyer EC, Kennedy GA: A new method of measuring diet abrasion and its effect on the development of the forestomach. J Dairy Sci. 1977;80:

2534-2541. DOI: 10.3168/jds.S0022-0302(97)76207-6

[29] Gelsinger SL, Coblentz WK, Zanton GI, Ogden RK, Akins MS: Physiological effects of starter-induced ruminal acidosis in calves before, during, and after weaning. J Dairy Sci. 2020;103:2762-2772. DOI: 10.3168/jds.2019-17494

[30] Bailey CB: Growth of digestive organs and their contents in holstein steers: Relation to body weight and diet. Can J Anim Sci. 1986;66:653-661. DOI: 10.4141/CJAS86-072

[31] Horvath KC, Miller-Cushon EK: Evaluating effects of providing hay on behavioral development and performance of group-housed dairy calves. J Dairy Sci. 2019;102:10411-10422. DOI: 10.3168/jds.2019-16533

[32] Mirzaei M, Khorvash M, Ghorbani GR, Kazemi-Bonchenari M, Ghaffari MH: Growth performance, feeding behavior, and selected blood metabolites of Holstein dairy calves fed restricted amounts of milk: No interactions between sources of finely ground grain and forage provision. J Dairy Sci. 2017;100:1086-1094 DOI: 10.3168/jds.2016-11592

[33] Barkema HW, von Keyserlingk MAG, Kastelic JP, Lam TJGM, Luby C, Roy JP, LeBlanc SJ, Keffe GP, Kelton DF: Invited review: Changes in the dairy industry affecting dairy cattle health and welfare. J Dairy Sci. 2015;98:7426-7445. DOI: 10.3168/JDS.2015-9377

[34] Martin NP, Russelle MP, Powell JM, Sniffen CJ, Smith SI, Tricarico JM, Grant RJ: Invited review: Sustainable forage and grain crop production for the US dairy industry. J Dairy Sci. 2017;100:9479-9494. DOI: 10.3168/JDS.2017-13080

[35] Halopka R: Hay market demand and price report for the Upper Midwest. UW-Madison Clark County Extension. 2021. Available from: http://fyi.uwex.edu/forage/ [Accessed 2021-03-09]

[36] Mirzaei M, Khorvash M, Ghorbani GR, Kazemi-Bonchenari M, Riasi A, Nabipour A, van den Borne JJGC: Effects of supplementation level and particle size of alfalfa hay on growth characteristics and rumen development in dairy calves. J Anim Physiol Anim Nutr (Berl). 2015;99:553-564. DOI: 10.1111/JPN.12229

[37] Kargar S, Kanani M, Albenzio M, Caroprese M: Substituting corn silage with reconstituted forage or nonforage fiber sources in the starter diets of Holstein calves: effects on performance, ruminal fermentation, and blood metabolites. J Anim Sci. 2019;97:3046-3055. DOI: 10.1093/JAS/SKZ180

[38] Kargar S, Kanani M: Reconstituted versus dry alfalfa hay in starter feed diets of Holstein dairy calves: Effects on feed intake, feeding and chewing behavior, feed preference, and health criteria. J Dairy Sci. 2019;102:4061-4071. DOI: 10.3168/JDS.2018-15189

[39] Beiranvand H, Khani M, Omidian S, Ariana M, Rezvani R, Ghaffari MH: Does adding water to dry calf starter improve performance during summer. J Dairy Sci. 2016;99:1903-1911. DOI: 10.3168/JDS.2015-10004

[40] Beiranvand H, Khani M, Ahmadi F, Omidi-Mirzaei H, Ariana M, Bayat AR: Does adding water to a dry starter diet improve calf performance during winter. Animal. 2019;13:959-967. DOI: 10.1017/S1751731118002367

[41] Felton CA, DeVries TJ: Effect of water addition to a total mixed ration on feed temperature, feed intake, sorting behavior, and milk production of dairy cows. J Dairy Sci. 2010;93:2651-2660. DOI: 10.3168/JDS.2009-3009

[42] Webb LE, Jensen MB, Engel B, van Reenen CG, Gerrits WJJ, de Boer IJM,

Bokkers EAM: Chopped or long roughage: what do calves prefer? Using cross point analysis of double demand functions. Plos One. 2014;9:e88778. DOI: 10.1371/journal.pone.0088778

[43] Omidi-Mirzaei H, Azarfar A, Mirzaei M, Kiani A, Ghaffari MH: Effects of forage source and forage particle size as a free-choice provision on growth performance, rumen fermentation, and behavior of dairy calves fed texturized starters. J Dairy Sci. 2018;101:4143-4157. DOI: 10.3168/jds.2017-13990

[44] Hill TM, Suarez-Mena FX, Dennis TS, Quigley JD, Schlotterbeck RL: Effects of free-choice hay on intake and growth of Holstein calves fed a textured starter to 2 months of age. Applied Animal Science. 2019;35:161-168. DOI: 10.15232/aas.2018-01826

[45] Ferraretto LF, Shaver RD, Luck BD: Silage review: Recent advances and future technologies for whole-plant and fractionated corn silage harvesting. J Dairy Sci. 2018;101:3937-3951. DOI: 10.3168/JDS.2017-13728

[46] Maulfair DD, Fustini M, Heinrichs AJ: Effect of varying total mixed ration particle size on rumen digesta and fecal particle size and digestibility in lactating dairy cows. J Dairy Sci. 2011;94:3527-3536. DOI: 10.3168/JDS.2010-3718

[47] Ferraretto LF, Shaver RD: Meta-analysis: Effect of corn silage harvest practices on intake, digestion, and milk production by dairy cows. Prof Anim Sci. 2012;28:141-149. DOI: 10.15232/S1080-7446(15)30334-X

[48] Montoro C, Miller-Cushon EK, DeVries TJ, Bach A: Effect of physical form of forage on performance, feeding behavior, and digestibility of Holstein calves. J Dairy Sci. 2013;96:1117-1124. DOI: 10.3168/jds.2012-5731

[49] Huhtanen P, Jaakkola S: The effects of forage preservation method and proportion of concentrate on digestion of cell wall carbohydrates and rumen digesta pool size in cattle. Grass Forage Sci. 1993;48:155-165. DOI: 10.1111/j.1365-2494.1993.tb01848.x

[50] Jaakkola S, Huhtanen P: The effects of forage preservation method and proportion of concentrate on nitrogen digestion and rumen fermentation in cattle. Grass Forage Sci. 1993;48:146-154. DOI: 10.1111/j.1365-2494.1993.tb01847.x

[51] Kehoe SI, Dill-McFarland KA, Breaker JD, Suen G: Effects of corn silage inclusion in preweaning calf diets. J Dairy Sci. 2019;102:4131-4137. DOI: 10.3168/jds.2018-15799

[52] Mirzaei M, Khorvash M, Ghorbani GR, Kazemi-Bonchenari M, Riasi A, Soltani A, Moshiri B, Ghaffari MH: Interactions between the physical form of starter (mashed versus textured) and corn silage provision on performance, rumen fermentation, and structural growth of Holstein calves. J Anim Sci. 2016;94:678-686. DOI: 10.2527/jas.2015-9670.

[53] Overvest MA, Bergeron R, Haley DB, DeVries TJ: Effect of feed type and method of presentation on feeding behavior, intake, and growth of dairy calves fed a high level of milk. J Dairy Sci. 2016;99:317-327. DOI: 10.3168/JDS.2015-9997

[54] Suarez BJ, Van Reenen CG, Stockhofe N, Dijkstra J, Gerrits WJJ: Effect of roughage source and roughage to concentrate ratio on animal performance and rumen development in veal calves. J Dairy Sci. 2007;90:2390-2403. DOI: 10.3168/jds.2006-524

[55] Block E, Shellenberger PR: Woodpulp fines of corn silage as roughages in complete rations or a pelleted complete ration for young dairy replacements from birth through 18 weeks of age. J Dairy Sci. 1980;63:2060-2070. DOI: 10.3168/JDS.S0022-0302(80)83183-3

[56] McDonald AP, Henderson R, Heron JE. The biochemistry of silage. 2nd ed. Marlow, England: Chalcombe; 1991 340 p.

[57] Cangiano LR, Yohe TT, Steele MA, Renaud DL: Invited Review: Strategic use of microbial-based probiotics and prebiotics in dairy calf rearing. Appl Anim Sci. 2020;36:630-651. DOI: 10.15232/AAS.2020-02049

[58] Xu S, Yang J, Qi M, Smiley B, Rutherford W, Wang Y, McAllister TA: Impact of Saccharomyces cerevisiae and Lactobacillus buchneri on microbial communities during ensiling and aerobic spoilage of corn silage. J Anim Sci. 2019;97:1273-1285. DOI: 10.1093/JAS/SKZ021

[59] Casper DP, Hultquist KM, Acharya IP: *Lactobacillus plantarum* GB LP-1 as a direct-fed microbial for neonatal calves. J Dairy Sci. 2021;104:5557-5568. DOI: 10.3168/JDS.2020-19438

[60] Ginane C, Baumont R, Favreau-Peigné A: Perception and hedonic value of basic tastes in domestic ruminants. Phys Behav. 2011;104:666-674. DOI: 10.1016/jphysbeh.2011.07.011

[61] Miller-Cushon EK, Montoro C, Ipharraguerre IR, Bach A: Dietary preference in dairy calves for feed ingredients high in energy and protein. J Dairy Sci. 2014;97:1634-1644. DOI: 10.3168/jds.2013-7199.

[62] de Passillé AM, Rushen J: What components of milk stimulate sucking in calves. Appl Anim Behav Sci. 2006;101:243-252. DOI: 10.1016/J.APPLANIM.2006.02.010

[63] National Animal Health Monitoring System(NAHMS). Dairy 2014: Dairy Cattle Management Practices in the United States, 2014. Available from: https://www.aphis.usda.gov/animal_health/nahms/dairy/downloads/dairy14/Dairy14_dr_PartI.pdf [Accessed 2021-03-15]

[64] Hill TM, Bateman HG, Aldrich JM, Quigley JD, Schlotterbeck RL: Evaluation of ad libitum acidified milk replacer programs for dairy calves. J Dairy Sci. 2013;96:3153-3162. DOI: 10.3168/JDS.2012-6132

[65] Provenza FD: Postingestive feedback as an elementary determinant of food preference and intake in ruminants. J Range Manag. 1995;48:2-17. DOI: 10.2307/4002498

[66] Ghassemi-Nejad J, Torbatinejad N, Naserian AA, Kumar S, Kim JD, Song YH, Ra CS, Sung KI: Effects of processing of starter diets on performance, nutrient digestibility, rumen biochemical parameters and body measurements of Brown Swiss dairy calves. Asian Australas J Anim Sci. 2012;25:980-987. DOI: 10.5713/AJAS.2011.11457

[67] Kanani M, Kargar S, Zamiri MJ, Ghoreishi SM, Mirzaei M: Reciprocal combinations of alfalfa hay and corn silage in the starter diets of Holstein dairy calves: effects on growth performance, nutrient digestibility, rumen fermentation and selected blood metabolites. Animal. 2019;13:2501-2509. DOI: 10.1017/S1751731119000934

[68] Zanton GI, Heinrichs AJ: Rumen digestion and nutritional efficiency of dairy heifers limit-fed a high forage ration to four levels of dry matter intake. J Dairy Sci. 2008;91:3579-3588. DOI: 10.3168/JDS.2008-1210

[69] Zanton GI, Heinrichs AJ: Digestion and nitrogen utilization in dairy heifers limit-fed a low or high forage ration at four levels of nitrogen intake. J Dairy Sci. 2009;92:2078-2094. DOI: 10.3168/JDS.2008-1712

[70] Pasha TN, Prigge EE, Russell RW, Bryan WB: Influence of moisture content of forage diets on intake and digestion by sheep. J Anim Sci. 1994;72:2455-2463. DOI:10.2527/1994.7292455x

[71] Baldwin RL, McLeod KR, Klotz JL, Heitmann RN: Rumen development, intestinal growth and hepatic metabolism in the pre- and postweaning ruminant. J Dairy Sci. 2004;87:E55-E65. DOI: 10.3168/JDS.S0022-0302(04)70061-2

[72] Górka P, Kowalski ZM, Zabielski R, Guilloteau P: *Invited review:* Use of butyrate to promote gastrointestinal tract development in calves. J Dairy Sci. 2018;101:4785-4800. DOI: 10.3168/jds.2017-14086

[73] Nemati M, Amanlou H, Khorvash M, Mirzaei M, Moshiri B, Ghaffari MH: Effect of different alfalfa hay levels on growth performance, rumen fermentation, and structural growth of Holstein dairy calves. J Anim Sci. 2016;94:1141-1148. DOI: 10.2527/JAS.2015-0111

[74] National Research Council. Nutrient requirements of dairy cattle (7th rev). Natl. Acad. Sci. Washington, D.C. 2001.

[75] Gerlach K, Roß F, Weiß K, Buscher W, Sudekum KH: Changes in maize silage fermentation products during aerobic deterioration and effects on dry matter intake by goats. Agric Food Sci. 2013;22:168-181. DOI: 10.23986/afsci.6739

[76] Bernardes TF, Daniel JLP, Adesogan AT, McAllister TA, Drouin P, Nussio LG, Huhtanen P, Tremblay GF, Belanger G, Cai Y: Silage Review: Unique challenges of silages made in hot and cold regions. J Dairy Sci. 2018;101:4001-4019. DOI: 10.3168/jds.2017-13703

[77] Pereira CS, Cunha SC, Fernandes JO: Prevalent mycotoxins in animal feed: Occurrence and analytical methods. Toxins (Basel). 2019;11:290. DOI: 10.3390/toxins11050290

[78] Nayakwadi S, Ramu R, Sharma AK, Gupta VK, Rajukumar K, Kumar V, Shirahatti PS, L Rashmi, Basalingappa KM: Toxicopathological studies on the effects of T-2 mycotoxin and their interaction in juvenile goats. PLOS One. 2020;15:e0229463. DOI: 10.1371/journal.pone.0229463

Chapter 9

Bromatological Analysis of the Fodder Marketed in the Peri-Urban Areas of Bujumbura (Burundi): Towards Spontaneous Fodder Conservation by Transformation into Silage

Joseph Butore, Daniel Sindaye, Mathias Hitimana, Jacques Nkengurutse and Tatien Masharabu

Abstract

Peri-urban areas of Bujumbura host a significant number of dairy cattle, which consequently ensure a substantial production of milk consumed in the Burundian capital. The presence of these cows in peri-urban areas has led to the emergence of an atypical market for spontaneous forage species. The present study seeks to determine the food and nutritional value of this fodder. A test on its conservation by transformation into silage was also carried out. Botanical field investigations and plant samples collection were carried out under the guidance of fodders suppliers. Based on the bromatological value deficiency thresholds for cattle, the results showed that the content of digestible nitrogenous matter and major elements (Ca, P, K, and Mg) in the forage is within acceptable limits. The final product obtained after fermentation, based on its color, its smell, and its consistency, is indeed silage. The chemical composition of fermented fodder showed that the nutritional quality has remained almost the same. Further research on digestibility of this forage is necessary. A study of the environmental determinants of spontaneous forage distribution at multiple sites and over a wide range of parameters may contribute to a better understanding of the importance of this fodder particularly in times of fodder deficit.

Keywords: Anaerobic fermentation, animal feed, floristic composition, forage, silo

1. Introduction

Buringa and Maramvya localities in peri-urban neighbourhoods of Bujumbura City (Burundi) house many dairy cow heads. Therefore, this ensures a significant production of milk consumed in the Burundian economic capital. In the past, this breeding was practiced either in the capital Bujumbura, in the Rusizi National Park -Palm Area (Rukoko), or other areas surrounding Bujumbura. As a result of the administrative and environmental protection measures, these cows have been moved to the peri-urban areas of Bujumbura, where it is sometimes difficult to find enough and sustainable feed for livestock.

The presence of these cows in the peri-urban areas of Bujumbura has led to the creation of a market for forage species to feed these animals. The reasons for the set-up of this new type of market include the fact that along the Rusizi River is the Rusizi National Park, where it is strictly forbidden to graze the herds, the proximity to Melchior Ndadaye International Airport, and plots of the Regional Development Corporation of Imbo (SRDI) for rice growing, etc.

This market system addresses the problem of grazing. It is so new and unusual in Burundi. However, it is a business that sustains the livelihood of a Sample of people and contributes to the development of the country. It is with this business that the city of Bujumbura is supplied (in part) with milk. However, the food and nutritional value of these plant species need to be documented as well as the socio-economic aspects of this trade.

Indeed, it is only in the peri-urban areas of the city of Bujumbura, where this type of business exists while livestock farming is practiced throughout the country. Again, those who trade are not native to the region in question. They come from different provinces of the country including Ngozi with a workforce of about 68% of sellers of this forage market of Buringa [1]. Thus, the present study seeks to determine the nutritional value of these fodders through an analysis of their bromatological value, firstly. Secondly, spontaneous fodder marketed at the Buringa market having already been described and characterized [2], their regular use confirmed by local breeders [1]. In addition, a test on their conservation by transformation into silage was also carried out in this study with a view to improve animal feed, and above all contributing to the sustainable use of this spontaneous fodder.

The socio-economic aspects of this new type of livestock and trade will be addressed in other publications.

2. Material and methods

2.1 Material

2.1.1 Study area

2.1.1.1 Buringa and Maramvya areas

The exploratory study was conducted at the Buringa fodder market (**Figure 1**) in the peri-urban area of Bujumbura. The sampling of forage plants studied has been carried out in the Buringa and Maramvya areas, located in Gihanga commune of Bubanza province, and Mutimbuzi commune of Bujumbura province. **Figure 2** showing the sampling area was generated using the QGIS Desktop 2.18.11 software. These areas are crossed by the National Road Nr 5 (RN 5). A seven-kilometer distance separates Melchior Ndadaye International Airport from the Buringa Forage Market. They are all part of the Imbo Plain [3]. The natural region of Imbo is characterized by a low altitude of about 1000 m and warm weather. This region is made up of the plain of Rusizi and the coastal plain of Lake Tanganyika. It is between $2^0$45 'and $4^0$27' South latitude and 29^0 and $39^0$40′ East longitude. The plain is bounded by two major horsts: the watershed of the Basins of the Congo and the Nile and the Itombwe massif, which borders the plain to the west in DR Congo. These mountains peak respectively at 2600 m and 3200 m of altitude. This particular situation, in an overheated basin and the south-east trade wind that crosses it further accentuates the semi-arid climate that characterizes it [4].

DOI: http://dx.doi.org/10.5772/intechopen.98217

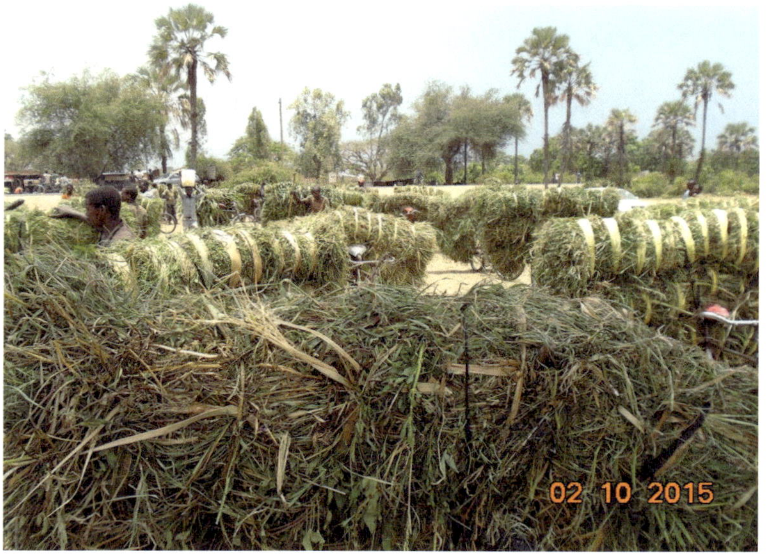

Figure 1.
Partial view of Buringa fodder market located in Gihanga commune of Bubanza province, Burundi.

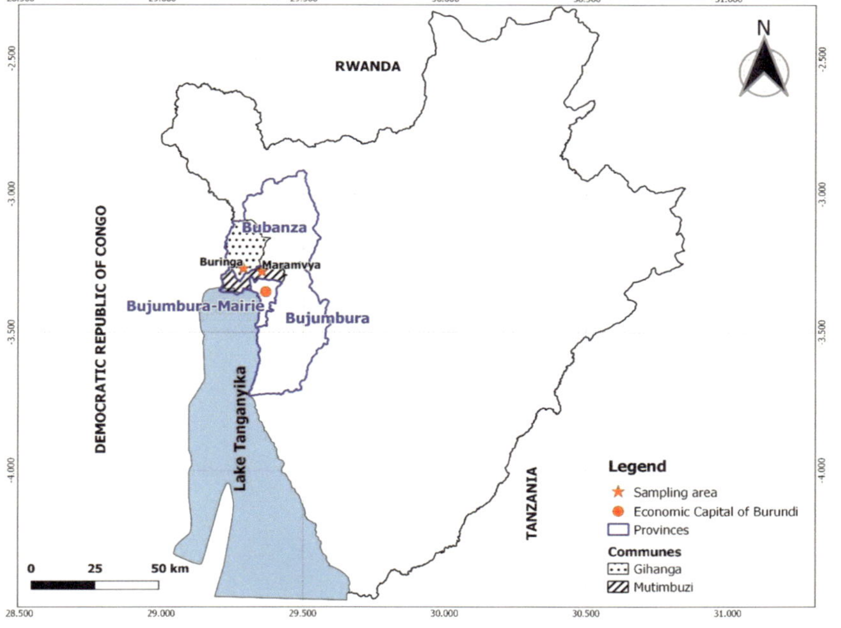

Figure 2.
Location of Buringa and Maramvya fresh fodder markets, located respectively in Gihanga commune of Bubanza province, and Mutimbuzi commune of Bujumbura province, Burundi.

2.1.1.2 Nyabunyegeri pisty and its facilities

The pigsty (**Figure 3**) in which the spontaneous anaerobic fodder fermentation experiment was carried out is on Nyabunyegeri hill in Mutimbuzi commune. This pigsty started its activities in 2016 and during our stay, it had around 150 pigs divided into different categories (suckling sows, gestating sows, empty sows, growing piglets, fattening pigs and boars).

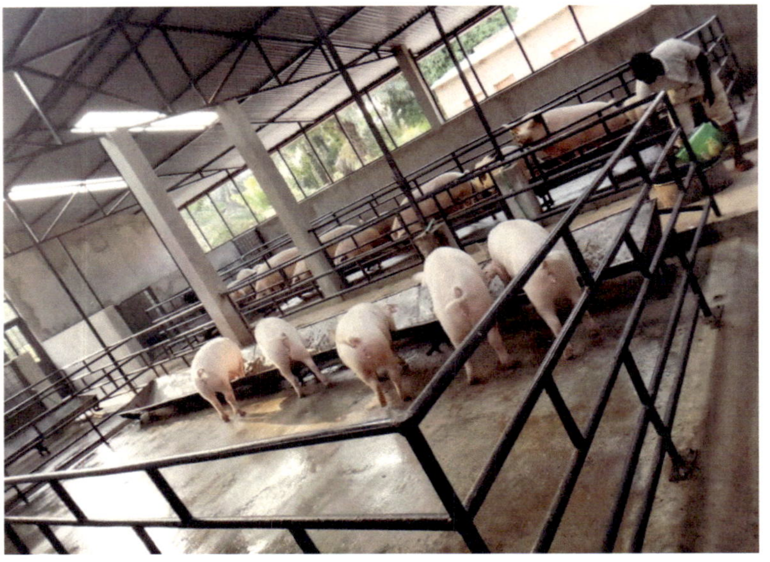

Figure 3.
Partial view of Nyabunyegeri pisty, Burundi.

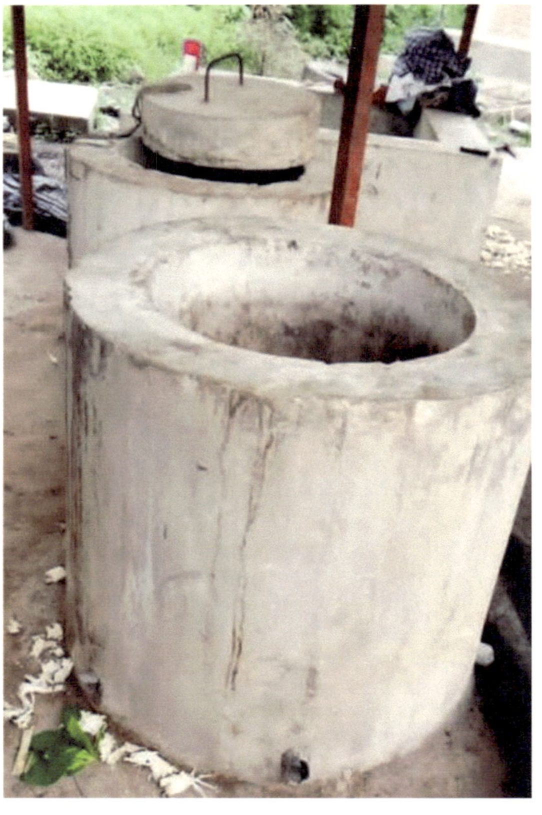

Figure 4.
The silo used during the experiment at Nyabunyegeri pigsty, Burundi.

The Nyabunyegeri pigsty has a few silos that are regularly used for anaerobic fermentation of herbs, wastes of seasonal fruits and other vegetables used in animal feed. One of these silos was used for our experiment (**Figure 4**).

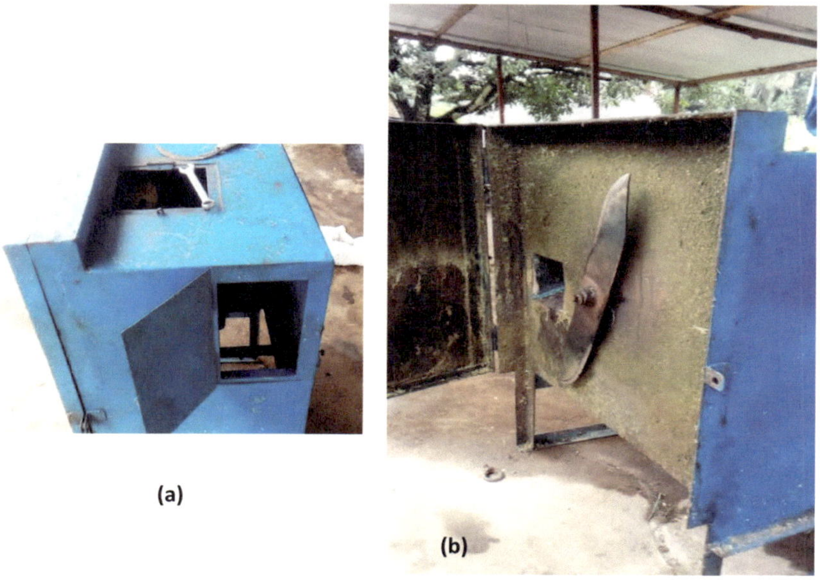

Figure 5.
Partial view of the chopping machine brand ITARA-M 9186/BI. (a) Outside view and (b) Chainsaw part.

The silo has a cylindrical shape with 0.5 m internal diameter; 0.6 m high with an almost smooth internal wall where there was no need to use cling film to ensure waterproofing except for the roof; volume 11.775,000 Cm^3. All parts of the silo are made of reinforced concrete, with a cylindrical wall 11 Cm thick; a heavy and circular cover which properly close the walls. The base of this small structure, but whose dimensions are well adapted to this type of experiment, was equipped with a few small pipes allowing the effluent to be released to the outside of the silo.

In the pigsty, the fodder chopping is carried out using a chopping machine brand ITARA- M 9186/BI (**Figure 5**) manufactured by young burundians grouped together in a cooperative called Cooperative of Innovation and Reflection for Integrated Development (CIRDI: Coopérative d'Innovation et de Réflexion pour le Développement Intégré).

2.1.2 Other material used

A bicycle for the transport of the fodder to be fermented (**Figure 6**), cooking salt (NaCl), molasses from sugar cane produced by the Mosso Sugar Factory (SOSUMO) located in Eastern Burundi in the Province of Rutana, 16 piglets in growth aged three months on which palatability was tested, and a camera.

The following equipment was used for the various analyzes carried out at the Agricultural Chemistry Laboratory of the Institute of Agronomic Sciences of Burundi (ISABU):

- The humidity/dry matter (crude and analytical) was analyzed with the following devices: analytical balance to within 1/10,000, an oven set at 105°, an appropriate crucible;

- The total ash at 600°C was determined using: an analytical balance, a porcelain capsule, an oven set at 600°C.

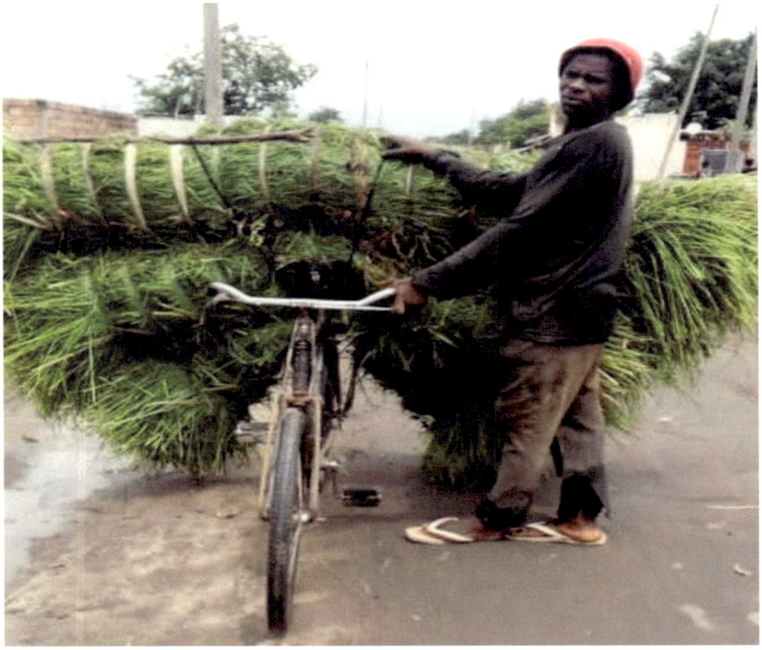

Figure 6.
Three bunches (batches) of a mixture of fresh fodder used for fodder conservation test by transformation into silage.

- The quantity of total phosphate was calculated using the following device: a mineralizer, U.V-visible.
- The protein contents were analyzed using: nitrogen mineralizer (Kjeldahl), Kjeldahl tube, digital burette, nitrogen still.
- The minerals Ca, Mg and K were calculated using: mineralizer, SSA, analytical balance.
- Crude cellulose (fibers) was analyzed using as devices: a hot plate, a refrigerator, a fiber extractor, an analytical balance.
- An analytical balance and a separating funnel were used for the analysis of the fat.

2.2 Methodology

2.2.1 Floristic composition and bromatological value

Collection of forage samples was made in the Buringa Zone of Gihanga Commune in Bubanza Province and the Maramvya Zone of Mutimbuzi Commune in Bujumbura Province under the guidance of fodders suppliers. The collection of samples can be described as follows: with the guide (a seller), we walked and when we arrived at the site of collection, he cut the grass as usual and put them at our disposal. Then, we reviewed all the species constituting the sample he handed to us. We took a small pile of 150–200 grams which was later subjected to analysis of the bromatological value. Three sites considered for having a relative high production of forage marketed in the fodder market had attracted our attention. These sites

DOI: http://dx.doi.org/10.5772/intechopen.98217

were rice plots, Mpanda cemetery and its surroundings, and the level curves. In each site, three forage samples were collected at different localities and in total nine forages samples were taken for bromatological analysis.

The database of flowering plants of tropical Africa [5] put online by the Conservatory and Botanical Garden of the City of Geneva and South African National Biodiversity Institute, Pretoria (African Flowering Plants Database version 3.3.4, http://www.ville-ge.ch/musinfo/bd/cjb/africa/) was consulted to check the nomenclature of species and families.

The analyses of the bromatological value of the forage batches were carried out in the Soils and Agro-Food Products Analysis Laboratory (LASPA) of the ISABU. The parameters analysed as follows:

- raw dry matter (DM) in % and analytical DM in % was analyzed using the gravimetric method at 105°C.
- fat in % DM was analyzed using the gravimetric method (petroleum ether extraction).
- protein in % DM was analyzed using the standardized method (ISO 11261, Modified Kjeldahl method, volumetric assay.
- crude cellulose in % DM was analyzed using WEENDE method (gravimetric method, attack by acid + soda).
- phosphorus in mg/kg DM was analyzed using the vanado-molybolic complex method by Ultra-Violet spectrophotometry, after mineralization (dry and with acid).
- potassium in mg/kg DM, Calcium in mg/kg DM and Magnesium in mg/kg DM were analyzed with the spectrophotometric atomic absorption (SSA) /flame assay method after dry and acid mineralization.

Nine samples from nine different sites were analyzed.

2.2.2 Anaerobic fermentation of spontaneous forages at Nyabunyegeri pigsty

The sample used to carry out a test on the fodder conservation by transformation into silage consisted of 3 bunches of a mixture of fresh forages dominated by Poaceae. The fodder used for this test was bought at the Buringa market, and transported by bicycle to Nyabunyegeri hill in the neighboring Commune of Mutimbuzi in Bujumbura province where there is a pigsty with vertical silos within it, regularly used in the manufacture of silage. One of the silos was used to conduct this experiment.

The fodder chopping was carried out using a chopping machine brand ITARA- M 9186/BI.

It should be noted that the fodder used was fresh, therefore, purchased, chopped, and fermented on the same day. The chopper had been set to cut the forage into 1 cm segments to meet the chopping dimensions at this host farm.

Always to comply with the practices of the host pigsty, cooking salt and molasses (were added to the chopped forages before fermenting them. These two products were added with respective doses of 1 kg and 2 kg per 100 kg of chopped fodder. The salt and molasses were first mixed separately, before being gradually incorporated into the chopped fodder during the various stages of compaction when filling the silo.

The compaction was done gradually and in two complementary ways, always following the practices of this farm in the fermentation of plants for pigs. First, the farm workers dipped their feet in boots (carefully washed first) in the silo to pack the fodder to ferment, layer by layer, jumping on the chopped fodder. Then the heavy silo cover was used and placed on the top layers inside the silo as well; this is to have a perfect settlement, that i.e.to completely expel the air from the biomass in order to guarantee anaerobic fermentation. The same cover was put on the silo at the end to close it tightly with its content.

Once cut and mixed with the molasses + salt solution, a sample of the fodder was analyzed at the same laboratory of ISABU in order to assess the biochemical composition of this type of food before fermentation. Another sample was taken from the finished product to undergo the same analyzes in the same laboratory, with the same methods, in the aim of determining possible changes in nutritional value.

The metabolizable energy was calculated using a formula provided by the same laboratory:

$$\text{Metabolizable energy in Kcal / kg of dry matter} = 3951 + 54.4 \text{ x fat} - 88.7 \text{ x fibers} - 40.8 \text{x ash} \quad (1)$$

The palatability test [6, 7].was conducted on pigs since the test was carried out in a pigsty where animals were fed with similar feed (but made from other types of forages) and on a regular basis. Thus, 6 kg of chopped fodder was taken from the mass to be fermented and distributed to 16 piglets aged three months. Once the silage was ready, i.e. 3 days after storage and closing the silo, the palatability test was repeated on the same piglets.

2.2.3 Statistical analysis

In order to assess the degree of similarity of forage samples in terms of presence-absence of the species, a dendrogram (Cluster analysis) was subsequently generated using the MVSP 3.1 software (Multi-Variate Statistical Package) with the Jaccard coefficient [8].

One-way ANOVA following Duncan's multiple ranges test (SPSS programming toll, IBM SPSS. 25) was performed to test whether within the rice plots, Mpanda cemetery and its surroundings, and the level curves, the bromatological value of the batches of forage samples collected differ significantly.

3. Findings

3.1 Floristic composition of analyzed samples

The analysis of the bromatological value included 9 batches of samples gathered from 9 collection sites. These 9 batches consisted of 5 to 11 species each one; 20 species in total including two undetermined species. The Poaceae family has 15 species. The five remaining species are families of Commelinaceae (2), Convolvulaceae (1), Portulacaceae (1), and Euphorbiaceae (1). **Annex 1** shows the floristic composition of each batch which has been subject of a bromatological analysis. No species of the family of the Fabaceae were recorded and analyzed. *Commelina diffusa* L. (Commelinaceae) and *Leersia hexandra* Sw. (Poaceae) occur in almost all batches analysed. This could provide information on their relative abundance in the study area. **Figure** 7 illustrates the degree of similarity between the nine batches of forage

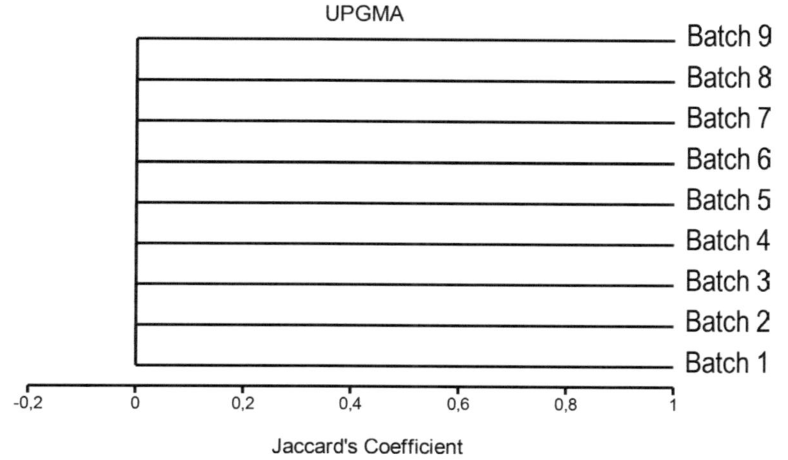

Figure 7.
Floristic affinities among the nine batches of forage samples collected in Buringa in Gihanga Commune and Maramvya in Mutimbuzi Commune (Burundi). Batch 1: Village 6 Gihanga, on rice dykes, Batch 2: Rubira/ Mpanda, Batch 3: Rukaramu- Mutimbuzi Commune, Batch 4: Gihanga-Rukoko 1, Batch 5: Gihanga-Rukoko 2, Batch 6: Mpanda Cemetery, Batch 7: in the premises of SRDI (Imbo Regional Development Corporation) headquarters, Batch 8: Rukaramu 2, Batch 9: Maramvya, on the edge of the irrigation canal of rice fields near a road.

samples in terms of presence-absence of species: there is no significant difference in terms of floristic composition.

3.2 Bromatological value of the fodder studied

The bromatological value of the fodder sold is not the same depending on their origin. The bromatological value analysis of the fodder is therefore very important for understanding its quality. The **Table 1** shows the nutrients composition of fodder from 3 different sites: rice plots, Mpanda cemetery and its surroundings, and the level curves. There was a significant difference ($p < 0.05$) both in crude fat and crude fiber. Likewise, none of the prospected sites produces a forage richer and more balanced in all nutrients compared to the other sites.

Item	Rice plots	Mpanda Cemetery	Level Curves	p-value
Crude DM %	78.11 ± 1.48	79.00 ± 1.64	77.33 ± 1.61	0.768
Analytical DM in %	94.08 ± 0.82	93.58 ± 0.73	94.26 ± 1.71	0.915
Crude Fat % in % DM	2.74 ± 0.12	2.64 ± 0.23	3.37 ± 0.98	0.03*
Crude Proteins % in % DM	18.09 ± 2.91	12.74 ± 1.22	17.04 ± 1.63	0.229
Crude fiber % in % DM	26.40 ± 0.68	28.69 ± 1.12	25.70 ± 0.42	0.085*
P in mg/kg DM	3144.66 ± 484.37	2860.00 ± 63.37	3034.33 ± 310.04	0.836
K in mg/kg DM	26156.33 ± 2905.08	29499.00 ± 2015.93	23057.00 ± 643.80	0.170
Ca in mg/kg DM	4246.33 ± 476.66	4925.66 ± 429.21	3950.00 ± 188.35	0.263
Mg in mg/kg DM	2403.33 ± 159.21	3519.33 ± 593.50	2483.00 ± 312.06	0.167

Table 1.
Bromatological value of the batches of forage samples collected at Buringa and Maramvya fresh fodder markets, respectively in Gihanga and Mutimbuzi Communes, Burundi based dry matter (DM) (DM: Dry Matter).

3.3 Food and nutritional value of spontaneous forage before and after anaerobic fermentation (direct silage)

The assessment of the food and nutritional value of the spontaneous fodder used was carried out in two stages: before and after anaerobic fermentation. **Figure 8** shows the forage ready to be fermented under anaerobic conditions; and **Figure 9** shows the forage resulting from the anaerobic fermentation. Initially, the forage was green in color. After fermentation, the color was yellow-brownish, a pleasant smell with a scent of molasses, and the fodder pieces separated easily from each other.

The results of the chemical composition analysis of the sample of fodder cut and mixed with the molasses + salt solution before fermentation, as well as that of another sample which was taken from the finished product (silage) is shown in **Table 2**.

3.4 Metabolizable energy

By applying the formula provided by ISABU, the metabolizable energy found for unfermented fodder was:

$$3951 + 54,4x1,84 - 88,7x32,5 - 40,8x11,5 = 699.146\,\text{kcal / kg of dry matter} \quad (2)$$

For fermented fodder, the metabolizable energy is as follows:

$$3951 + 54.4x1,26 - 88.7x26,9 - 40.8x17,2 = 931.754\,\text{kcal / kg of dry matter} \quad (3)$$

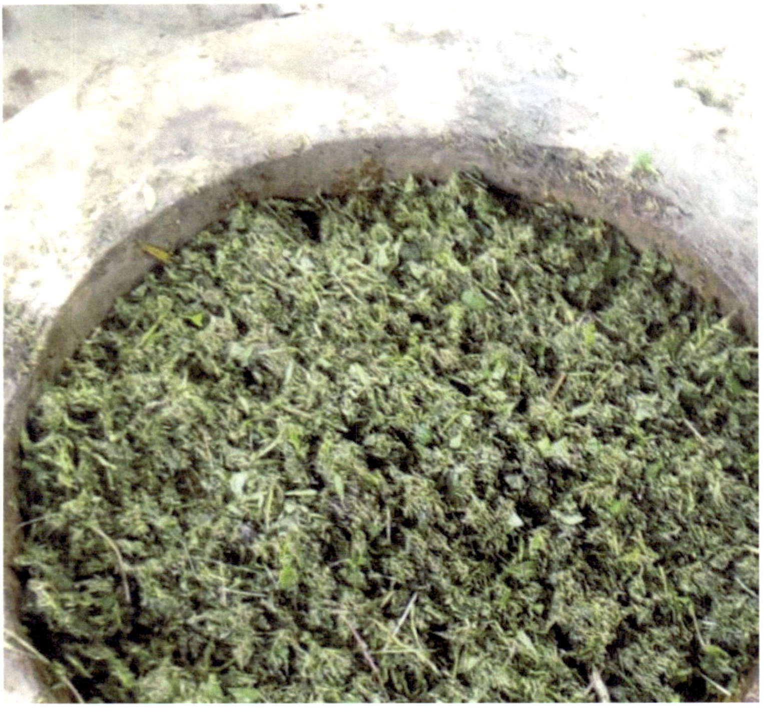

Figure 8.
Chopped fodder ready for fermentation.

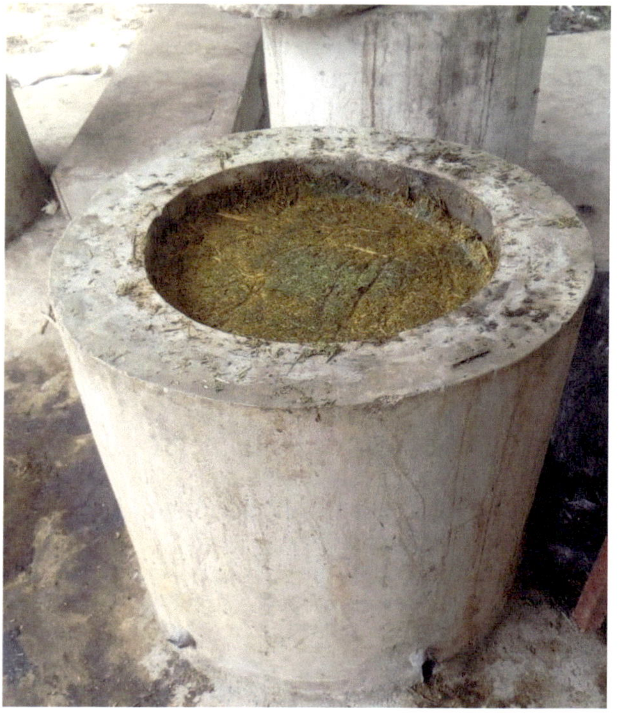

Figure 9.
Fermented fodder when the silo is opened (clearly visible brownish-yellow color).

Sample	Forage cut and mixed with the molasses + salt solution before fermentation	Final product after fermentation (Silage)
Laboratory Number	K 481	K 482
Raw Dry Matter (DM) %	24,2	22,7
Analytical DM in %,	98,4	97,9
Fat in % DM	1,84	1,26
Total ash in % DM	11,5	17,2
Proteins in % DM	7,73	8,44
Crudes fibers in % DM	32,5	26,9
Magnesium in mg/kg DM.	2660	2513
Calcium in mg/kg DM	2891	8864
Potassium in mg/kg DM	25104	19374
Total Phosphorus in mg/kg DM	171	160

Table 2.
Chemical composition of a sample of forage cut and mixed with the molasses + salt solution before fermentation (K 481), as well as that of another sample that was taken from the finished product after fermentation (K 482). DM: Dry Matter.

3.5 Palatability test

The 6 kg of chopped fodder which was taken from the quantity to be fermented was completely consumed by 16 three-month-old piglets in 25 minutes. For the ready silage, i.e. 3 days after storage and closure of the silo, the same amount of feed was this time consumed by the 16 young pigs in 28 minutes. It should be noted that no discomfort was observed in any of these animals after consuming both types of feed, one from chopped fodder ready for fermentation, and the other from the silage itself.

4. Discussion

4.1 Floristic composition of forage samples

The degree of similarity among the nine samples of forage samples in terms of presence-absence of the species does not suggest a significant difference. However, the nutritional value of the forage sold is not the same (**Table 1**). The bromatological value of forages varies according to several parameters including the richness of the soil in fertile elements, the vegetative stage of the plant, and the mode of preservation of the fodder (fresh or preserved) [9].

Given that the consideration of several environmental variables is likely to increase the explained floristic variability [10, 11], a study of the environmental determinants of the distribution of spontaneous forages at several sites and on a varied range of parameters is to consider. In fact, in nature, environmental factors (biological, physical, historical, etc.) do not act in isolation: they can influence one another or in synergy. Other factors that are difficult to quantify and dissociate, such as climatic fluctuations, chance, mortality, inter-and intraspecific competition, predation, geographical barriers to the spread of plant diaspores, dispersal agents, substrate, etc. may also interfere [12].

4.2 Bromatological value of forage samples

It was observed a significant difference ($p < 0.05$) both in crude fat and crude fiber. Except Phosphorus (P) composition which is relatively high in rice plot and level curves, the forage from Mpanda cemetery and its surroundings had a relative high composition in Potassium (K) Calcium (Ca), and Magnesium (Mg). In line with that, many researches had shown many factors which are responsible for the spontaneous species nutritional value composition. These include soil factors, such as soil pH, available nutrients, soil texture, organic matter content and soil-water relationships, weather and climatic factors, the crop and cultivar, postharvest handling and storage, and fertilizer applications and cultural practices [13–17].

Based on the bromatological value deficiency thresholds for cattle, the results show that the content of digestible nitrogenous matter (DNM) and major elements (Ca, P, K, and Mg) in the forage is within acceptable limits. The mineral content is greater than 0.26% Ca, 0.18% P, 0.60% K and 0.10% Mg/kg DM, and the DNM content is greater than 25 g/kg of DM [18].

The specific differences observed in the indicators of the bromatological value of the fodder sold at the Buringa fodder market would be linked to the nature of the soil and to the activities taking place regularly on each site. But it should be noted that the average quantities found, indicator by indicator, fall within the range of biochemical standards for green feed for animals [19].

There is always compensation and supplementation. The farmers mix forage from different localities or associate them with some concentrates for livestock, which increases the fodder quality. Burundian breeders traditionally provide a mineral supplement to livestock from mostly the Imbo saline soils (Icuhiro) [20]. These salty soils can ultimately correct sodium deficiency and meet the calcium and magnesium requirements of livestock. Then, the deficiency in some mineral elements of the forage is compensated by these salty soils.

4.3 Assessment of the food and nutritional value of spontaneous fodder before and after fermentation (direct silage): towards fodder conservation by transformation into silage of spontaneous fodder

For the sample of unfermented spontaneous fodder, the data in **Tables 1** and **2** are very close. This is because the spontaneous fodder used came from the same region. After fermentation, a slight decrease was observed for the following indicators: dry matter, fat, raw fiber, Magnesium, and Phosphorus. A small increase was observed for protein.

The sound variations were observed for the total ash for which the content went from 11.5% to 17.2%; and Calcium, for which the quantity tripled from 2891 mg/kg of dry matter to 8864 mg/kg of dry matter. Similar changes in mineral content have also been reported by Agence Française de Sécurité Sanitaire des Aliments, AFSSA [21].

4.4 Metabolizable energy

The metabolizable energy found for unfermented forages was 699.146 kcal/kg of dry matter while for fermented fodder it was 931.754 kcal/kg of dry matter.

This increasing trend of metabolizable energy would be a combined consequence of mastering good storage conditions by fermentation, plus the influence of added silage agents (molasses).

But it should also be noted that growing piglets need more metabolizable energy [19] which our fermented fodder cannot provide on its own; hence the need to supplement it with other types of feeds more rich in energy.

4.5 Palatability

A relative decrease in appetite for fermented forage was observed in this study. This relative decrease in palatability is also mentioned by AFSSA [21] which specifies that with rare exceptions, the ingestibility of fodder stored as silage is lower than that of the corresponding green fodder. The 3-day waiting period after storage and closing the silo were considered to meet the time usually observed in this pigsty during the fermentation of fodder. It should be noted that no discomfort was observed in any of these animals after consuming both types of feed, one from the chopper fodder before fermentation and the other from the silage itself. It was this encouraging observation, moreover, that led us to distribute to the piglets the entire quantity of the fermented fodder up to the end. Finally, it should be noted that in comparison with the silage prepared previously in this pigsty, it is the one resulting from our experiment that the piglets ate more quickly, i.e. 6 kg in 28 minutes for 16 piglets against 31 minutes for the same quantity of silage, and the same number of growing piglets.

Our results on the palatability test are similar to those of other studies [22, 23] who confirmed that the aroma of molasses improves food consumption by swine species.

5. Conclusion

This study focused on the assessment of the bromatological value of the fodder traded in Buringa, in peri-urban areas of the city of Bujumbura, Burundi. A test on their conservation by transformation into silage was also carried out in this study with a view to improve animal feed, and above all contributing to the sustainable use of these fodder.

Given that from a qualitative point of view stating that the bromatological value of the fodder sold at the fodder market is not the same (DM, Protein, Fat, Mineral matter), it is possible for a breeder to choose a fodder supplier site for his livestock taking into account the specific needs of the animals.

It was observed that the fodder content in minerals is relatively high. This is explained by the fact that the soil of the Imbo plain is generally saline [20]. Finally, the overall quality of the fodder is good although the nutritional value of each forage species sold, and considered individually, has not been documented.

Organoleptically speaking, the final product obtained, based on its color, its smell and its consistency, is indeed silage. The chemical composition of the product (fermented fodder) indicates that the nutritional quality has remained almost the same. The stored food is well palatable by the animals. Finally, the conservation of spontaneous Buringa fodder by anaerobic fermentation makes feasible the sustainable use of this feed in the farm without compromising its food and nutritional value.

Further research on digestibility of this forage is necessary. Moreover, a study of the environmental determinants of spontaneous forage distribution at multiple sites and over a wide range of parameters may contribute to a better understanding of the importance of this fodder particularly in times of fodder deficit.

Acknowledgements

This study was conducted as part of the collaboration between the Department of Animal Production of the Faculty of Agronomy and Bio-Engineering and the Department of Biology of the Faculty of Sciences of the University of Burundi, through the "Animal Production in periurban zone and safeguarding a protected ecosystem in an anthropized landscape" Project. The authors would like to take this opportunity to express their heartfelt thanks to the University of Burundi for their support. Our sincere thanks also go to the local authorities of Buringa and Maramvya, the forage sellers, and the breeders for their collaboration during the fieldwork.

Annex 1:

Floristic composition of the nine batches of forage samples collected from Buringa in Gihanga Commune and Maramvya in Mutimbuzi Commune (Burundi), and subjected to bromatological analysis. These samples represent the forage traded in Buringa (+: Presence, −: Absence). Sample 1: Village 6 Gihanga, on rice dykes, Sample 2: Rubira/Mpanda, Sample 3: Rukaramu-Commune Mutimbuzi, Sample 4: Gihanga-Rukoko 1, Sample 5: Gihanga-Rukoko 2, Sample 6: Mpanda Cemetery, Sample 7: Sample 7: in the premises of SRDI (Imbo Regional Development Corporation) headquarters Sample 8: Rukaramu 2, Sample 9: Maramvya, on the edge of the irrigation canal of rice plots near a road.

Family	Species/Batch samples	1	2	3	4	5	6	7	8	9
Commelinaceae	*Commelina diffusa* L	+	+	+	—	+	—	+	+	+
	Commelina africana L.	—	—	—	+		+	—	—	—
Convolvulaceae	*Ipomoea aquatica* Forssk.	—	+	—	+	—	—	—	+	+
Euphorbiaceae	*Euphorbia sp.*	+	—	—	—	—	—		—	—
Portulacaceae	*Portulaca oleracea* L.	+	—	—	—		—	—	+	—
	Cynodon nlemfuensis Vanderyst	—	—	+	+	+	+	+	—	+
	Digitaria abyssinica (Hochst. ex A. Rich.) Stapf	—	—	—	—	—	+	—	—	—
	Echinochloa pyramidalis (Lam.) Hitchc. & Chase	—	—	—	+	—	—	—	—	—
	Eriochloa meyeriana (Nees) Pilg.	—	—	—	+	—	+	—		—
	Indet.1	—	—	+	—	+	—	+	—	—
	Indet.2	—	—	—	+	—	—	—	—	—
Poaceae	*Leersia hexandra* Sw.	+	+	+	+	+	—	+	+	+
	Oryza longistaminata A. Chev. & Roehr.	+	+	—	+	—	—		+	+
	Panicum maximun Jacq.	—	—	—	—	—	—	+	+	+
	Panicum trichocladum Hack. ex K. Schum.	—	—	—	+	+	+	+	—	—
	Paspalidium germinatum (Forssk.) Stapf	—	—	+	—	—	—	+	—	—
	Pennisetum purpureum Schumach.	—	+		+	—	—	—	—	—
	Pseudobromus silvaticus K. Schum.	—	—	—	—	+	+	—	—	—
	Setaria homonyma (Steud.) Chiov.	—	—	—	—	—	+	—	—	—
	Setaria longiseta P. Beauv.	—	—	—	+	+	+	—	—	—
Total	20	5	5	5	12	7	8	7	6	6

Author details

Joseph Butore[1], Daniel Sindaye[1,2], Mathias Hitimana[3,4], Jacques Nkengurutse[3] and Tatien Masharabu[3]*

1 Department of Health and Animal Productions, Faculty of Agronomy and Bio-Engineering, University of Burundi, Bujumbura, Burundi

2 South China Agricultural University, Maoming Branch, Guangdong Laboratory for Lingnan Modern Agriculture, Guangdong Provincial Key Laboratory of Animal Nutrition Control, National Engineering Research Center for Breeding Swine Industry, College of Animal Science, Guangzhou, China

3 Faculty of Sciences, Research Centre in Natural and Environmental Sciences, University of Burundi, Bujumbura, Burundi

4 School of Life Sciences, Key Laboratory for Geographical Process Analysis and Simulation, Central China Normal University, Hubei Province, Wuhan, China

*Address all correspondence to: tatien.masharabu@ub.edu.bi

References

[1] Sindaye D. Etude sur le commerce du fourrage dans la zone périurbaine de Bujumbura: cas des zones Buringa et Maramvya. Mémoire d'Ingénieur Agronome, Université du Burundi ; 2016.

[2] Masharabu T., Butore J., Sindaye D., Hitimana M. Diversité floristique et distribution potentielle des essences fourragères spontanées au Burundi. *Geo-Eco-Trop*; 2019: 43(1): 161-170.

[3] Ministère de la planification du développement et de la reconstruction nationale. Monographie des communes Gihanga et Mutimbuzi. Bujumbura-Burundi; 2006.

[4] Dewez J. La culture cotonnière dans l'Imbo. ISABU, Bujumbura; 1986.

[5] Lebrun J.-P., Stork A.L. Enumération des plantes à fleurs d'Afrique tropicale et Tropical African Flowering Plants: *Ecology and Distribution*; 1991-2015: vol. 1-7. Conservatoire et Jardin botaniques de la Ville de Genève.

[6] Forbes J.M. Palatability: principles, methodology and practice for farm animals. *Animal Science Reviews* ; 2010 : 239-250 in CAB Reviews: Perspectives in Agriculture, Veterinary Science, Nutrition and Natural Resources; 2010: 5(052) : 1-15.

[7] Baumont R. Palatabilité et comportement alimentaire chez les ruminants. *INRA Production Animale*; 1996: 9 (5) : 349-358.

[8] Kovach W.L. MVSP: Multi-Variate Statistical Package data analysis.*Kovach Computing Services*; 85 Nant-y-Felin, Pentraeth, Anglesey; 1997.

[9] Diouf A. Typologie des exploitations et étude de rentabilité des cultures fourragères dans les systèmes de production du Bassin arachidier du Sénégal. Mémoire d'Ingénieur AgroEconomiste. Ecole Nationale Supérieure d'Agriculture de Thiès; 2002.

[10] Masharabu T. Flore et végétation du Parc National de la Ruvubu au Burundi: diversité, structure et implications pour la conservation. Editions Universitaires Européennes, Sarrebruck-Allemagne; 2012. 256 p.

[11] Masharabu T., Noret N., Bigendako M.J., Godart M.-F., Lejoly J., Bogaert, J. Effects of Fabaceae cover on soil parameters and analysis of environmental determinants of floristic variability in North-Eastern Ruvubu, Burundi. *International Journal of Current Trends in Science and Technology*; 2011: 2(2): 113-124.

[12] Lobo J.M., Castro I., Moreno J.C. Spatial and environmental determinants of vascular plant species richness distribution in the Iberian Peninsula and Balearic Islands. *Botanical Journal of the Linnean Society*; 2001: 73:233-253.

[13] Widdig M., Heintz-Buschart A., Schleuss P. M., Guhr A., Borer E. T., Seabloom E. W., Spohn M. Effects of nitrogen and phosphorus addition on microbial community composition and element cycling in a grassland soil. *Soil Biology & Biochemistry; 2020: 151.*

[14] Lenhart P. A. Using plant nutrient landscapes to assess Anthropocene effects on insect herbivores. *Current Opinion in Insect Science; 2017: 23*: 51-58.

[15] Waldrop M. P., Holloway J. M., Smith D. B., Goldhaber M. B., Drenovsky R. E., Scow K. M., Dick R., Howard D., Wylie B., Grace J. B. The interacting roles of climate, soils, and plant production on soil microbial communities at a continental scale. *Ecology; 2017: 98*(7): 1957-1967.

[16] Feng C. , Ai Y. , Chen Z. , Liu H., Wang K. , Xiao J. , Chen J., Huang Z.

Spatial variation of soil properties and plant colonisation on cut slopes: a case study in the semi-tropical hilly areas of China. *Plant Ecology & Diversity; 2016: 9*(1): 81-88.

[17] Moghadam F. S., Zimmer M. (2016). Effects of warming, nutrient enrichment and detritivore presence on litter breakdown and associated microbial decomposers in a simulated temperate woodland creek. *Hydrobiologia;2016: 770*(1): 243-256.

[18] Sikumbili V., Mandiki S. Teneurs en éléments majeurs, Calcium, Potassium, Magnésium et Phosphore et valeur fourragère (énergie-protéines) des pâturages naturels de la sous-région pastorale de l'Ituri (République du Zaïre). *Tropicultura*; 1989 :7 (4) : 158-163.

[19] Khokhrin S.N. Study guide for higher educational institutions in 310800 "Veterinary Medicine"/editor TS Molochaeva; Moscow, 2007. Ser. Textbooks and teaching aids for students of university.

[20] Gourdin J., Tilquin J.P., Hollebosch P., Kibiriti C. Icuhiro, complément minéral utilisé dans l'élevage traditionnel au Burundi. *Tropicultura* ; 1989 : 7(2) : 52-54.

[21] AFSSA. Bonnes pratiques de fabrication de l'ensilage pour une meilleure maîtrise des risques sanitaires. Rapport technique; 2004.

[22] Laitat M., De Jaeger F., Vandenheede M., Nicks B. Facteurs influençant la consommation alimentaire et les performances zootechniques du porc sevré : perception et caractéristiques de l'aliment. *Annales de Médecine Vétérinaire* ; 2004 : 148 : 15-29

[23] McLaughlin C.L., Baile C.A., Buckholtz L.L., Freeman S.K. Preferred flavours and performance of weanling pigs. *Journal of Animal Science* ; 1983 : 56 : 1287-1293.